THE
SEASONED
PSYCHOTHERAPIST

— Triumph Over Adversity —

Carl Goldberg, Ph. D.

W. W. Norton & Company
New York   London

Printed in the United States of America.

First Edition

The text of this book was composed in English Times. Composition by Bytheway
Typesetting Services, Inc. Manufacturing by Haddon Craftsmen, Inc.
Book design by Justine Burkat Trubey

Library of Congress Cataloging-in-Publication Data

Goldberg, Carl.
    The seasoned psychotherapist : triumph over adversity / Carl
Goldberg.
        p.   cm.
    Includes bibliographical references.
    ISBN 0-393-70146-8
    1. Psychotherapists—Psychology.   2. Psychotherapists—Mental
health.   3. Middle age—Psychological aspects.   4. Psychotherapy—
Vocational guidance.   I. Title.
    [DNLM: 1. Career Choice.   2. Middle Age—psychology.   3. Personal
Satisfaction.   4. Psychotherapy.   WM 420 G618s]
RC480.5.G586   1992
616.89′14′023—dc20
DNLM/DLC   92-16191   CIP
for Library of Congress

W.W. Norton & Company, Inc., 500 Fifth Avenue, New York, N.Y. 10110
W.W. Norton & Company, Ltd., 10 Coptic Street, London WC1A 1PU

1 2 3 4 5 6 7 8 9 0

THE
SEASONED
PSYCHOTHERAPIST

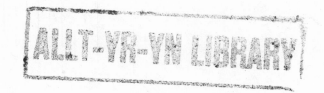

By the same author

Encounter

Therapeutic Partnership

The Human Circle

In Defense of Narcissism

On Being a Psychotherapist

Understanding Shame

Social System Perspectives in Residential Institutions
(with Howard W. Polsky and Daniel S. Claster)

The Dynamics of Residential Treatment
(with Howard W. Polsky and Daniel S. Claster)

Clinical Studies of Adult Development
(with Michael Commons and Jack Demick)

A Norton Professional Book

ACKNOWLEDGMENTS

I would like to express my gratitude to my wife, Virginia Crespo, M.S.W., Daniel Claster, Ph.D., Sandra Haber, Ph.D., my editor, Susan Barrows Munro, Richard C. Robertiello, M.D., and Myron Weiner, M.D., for their generous help and astute ideas for presenting the study reported in this book.

I also am deeply appreciative to the sixty-four seasoned practitioners who share their lives and practices with the reader and me.

CONTENTS

THE
SEASONED
PSYCHOTHERAPIST

— one —

INTRODUCTION:
BEHIND THE CONSULTING ROOM DOOR

> To everything there is a season,
> and a time to every purpose under the heavens.
> A time to be born and a time to die,
> A time to plant and a time to pluck that which is planted.
>
> — Ecclesiastes III, 1:2

For too long the lives of psychotherapists have remained hidden behind a mystique. Traditionally, books about psychotherapy discuss the theoretical ideas and clinical techniques of its practitioners. When these accounts examine the actual events of the consulting room, rarely do they purview in any illuminating way the impact that the therapist's personal life has upon what happens in the office; nor, for that matter, do they look at the effect of clinical practice on the therapist's private life.

The Seasoned Psychotherapist is a continuation of the examination of the lives of psychotherapists that I began in *On Being a Psychotherapist* (1986) and followed with *Understanding Shame* (1991). The major theme of these volumes was that, since the person and the practice of the psychotherapist are inexorably related, we need to be thoroughly aware of how the professional and personal aspects of the practitioner's life are interrelated in order to deepen our understanding of psychotherapeutic practice. *The Seasoned Psychotherapist* focuses on the issues of mature practice. There have been no previous professional books that in any concerted way addressed the

1

concerns and dilemmas of being an experienced practitioner of psychoanalysis or psychotherapy.*

Maturity is the time in our career when we can most wisely reflect
upon our own experience. I have been a psychotherapist for the past
twenty-five years. I have reached a point in my career and in my
personal life at which people generally begin to ask themselves some
vital questions about where they have come in their lives and what is
still realistically attainable in the time that they have left. This crucial
inquiry about how we will design our own life structure has to do
with the vital tasks of mid-life, which researchers into the developmental stages of adulthood have told us each person has to undergo
in order appropriately to direct one's life toward the requirements of
constructive maturity.

In reflecting on my life and professional career, I wondered what
other experienced practitioners have had to report about how the
developmental issues of mid-life and the years beyond have affected
their lives and practices. For example, in what ways have they found
their daily existence to be subjectively and qualitatively different
from that of a younger and less experienced person?

Extensively searching the psychological literature on the lives and
practices of mature practitioners, I found no empirical data or any
substantial research on how psychotherapists handle the issues of
mid-life and the years beyond. It is curious that a profession which
purportedly holds empirical behavioral research in the highest regard
has not scientifically investigated the subject of practitioner maturity,
which is of crucial direct consequence to the therapist and has significant indirect impact on patients' lives.

Actually, my own need to have a perspective from which to view
and understand my own mid-career issues would be addressed by
even a few insightful self-reports from highly articulate and wise
senior practitioners. I would ask them whether they thought mature
therapists are like other mature people who are not practitioners of
healing. Their personal accounts would help to answer the central
questions that I have tried to address in this book: Do mature psychotherapists face the same developmental concerns as other people or
do they have unique issues? and Does being a well trained and experi-

---

*Who the "seasoned" practitioner is cannot be calculated by simply the number of
years of clinical practice. Each practitioner will phenomenologically experience his
or her therapeutic maturity in his or her own particular way. Generally, however, we
can operationally define the experienced therapist as someone who has had a
serious commitment to being a practitioner for at least a decade.

enced examiner of the human psyche enable seasoned practitioners to live richer, wiser, and more mature lives than they would have been capable of living had they not become psychotherapists?

These questions would seem to be the kinds of inquiry thoughtful practitioners would periodically ask themselves in trying to understand their relationship to their patients. Nevertheless, my search of the psychological and psychoanalytic literature unearthed few personal vignettes, or even statements, about how mature practitioners have dealt with these life issues.

What I found to be the most astounding, as a result of my search, was that the largest source of information about the lives of experienced practitioners was to be found in popular literature rather than in social science publications. The impression that these popular accounts give about the practice and personal character of psychotherapists is almost entirely virulent. Many of these short stories and novels appear to be thinly disguised accounts of the author's personal experience as a patient with a therapist who is presented as undergoing a personal crisis or as bedeviled by some unusual abnormality; the stress or deviance leads the therapist to commit questionable or unethical behavior with patients. The best know of these stories is F. Scott Fitzgerald's *Tender Is the Night*.

A few senior practitioners have themselves written novels about the practice of psychotherapy. The best of these are the novels of Allen Wheelis, an eminent San Francisco psychoanalyst, who portrays the perils of mature therapeutic practice in his *The Doctor of Desire* and *The Seeker*.

The literature on psychotherapeutic practice compels the experienced practitioner to walk alone in the night. It gives the unmistakable impression that the vast material on examining therapeutic practice focuses almost exclusively on understanding the neophyte practitioner. Yet the task of maturation is continuous, never finally secured. Each stage of life imposes new demands and reexamination of previous satisfactions and life solutions. Nonetheless, those who write on the subjects of psychoanalysis and psychotherapy have made the tacit assumption that once the practitioner acquires clinical skills he or she should be able to maintain them with facility over a lifetime (Goldberg, 1990b). Those who make this assumption serve their colleagues poorly. We can no longer afford as senior practitioners to disregard the process of *disillusionment* that comes through aging and maturation, a troubling disillusionment that has seriously afflicted a considerable number of practitioners — if not every practitioner—of psychotherapy at some point in the senior years of practice.

Clearly, serious dissatisfactions in one's practice and private life will reduce clinical effectiveness. But no less significantly, it will concomitantly jeopardize the practitioner's physical, emotional, and spiritual well-being (Goldberg, 1990b). Each vocational career has its limitations and its own particular perils. However, there are some careers that are at times downright dangerous. The practice of psychotherapy is one of these. The work we are involved in has profound effects upon our health and well-being.

Perhaps the reason that a book like this has not been written before is that the subject is one about which we as practitioners know the least—how to take care of ourselves. Neither in our course work nor in our clinical training are we taught the necessary skills for coping with our own stress. Yet we flood the market with books and articles on how to treat the conflicts of our patients. We may be our own most difficult patients. The very significant rates among senior practitioners of "burn-out," deep depression, broken relationships and suicide attest to the difficulties that many experienced practitioners have in coming to terms with the developmental issues of maturity.

As senior practitioners we might profit by having the mentoring of inspired role models as we face the necessary developmental issues of mature practice. As we mature we shed certain illusions and some of us enter a wiser and more authentic way of being. The question is why some practitioners have evolved to a higher plane of being, while others have not.

Unfortunately, our profession has fostered a mystique. As a result of the uniform unwillingness of experienced practitioners to supply information about themselves, we know less about the lives of psychotherapists than about any other prominent profession (Henry, Sims, & Spray, 1973). It would only be a slight exaggeration to submit that seasoned practitioners know little more about the issues of mature practice than what has actually happened in their own lives and practices. We probably know more about the private lives of our accountant, attorney and physician than we do about our own colleagues.

As psychotherapists we recognize that the serious personal issues of practice require open and frank discussion; yet there is also, as Burton (1972) indicated in his book about the lives of therapists, "a natural repugnance in man that militates against revealing the innermost details of his life" (p. 186). This reluctance about self-revelation is supported by the scholarly tradition that maintains that the personal aspects of the life of the scientist or practitioner have no place in professional, let alone popular, publications. This state of affairs represents the model offered to us by Sigmund Freud. In the Introduction to volume III of Ernest Jones's (1961) biography of Freud we are informed:

> On several occasions Sigmund Freud expressed himself strongly against being made the subject of biographical study, giving it as one of his reasons that the only important thing about him was his ideas — his personal life, he said, could not be of the slightest concern to the world. (p. vii)

Freud was mistaken in his disregard of the biography of the psychotherapist. The obscurity of the private life that he endorsed has furnished an unfortunate concealment behind which practitioners (perhaps overly concerned that their patients would be adversely affected by learning intimate details about their therapist's life) have remained hidden. However, if the findings of my study of mature practice accurately represent current psychotherapy, it would appear that the healing endeavor is becoming an increasingly less secretive process. Hopefully, in bringing into the open experienced practitioners' personal concerns, this volume will help to promote a greater understanding of psychotherapeutic practice by providing illumination on the men and women who are involved in the task of healing the wounds of the human psyche.

THE AUTHOR'S PERSPECTIVE

I did not write this book as an expert on taking care of myself, as I might about treating difficult patients. I have written as a practitioner who has thought seriously about the issues of midlife maturity and has access to the self-reports of other seasoned practitioners about their struggles in coming to terms with maturity. These struggles were reported to me by questionnaires and face-to-face in-depth interview. Chapters 5 and 7 report the findings of my research on the lives of mature practitioners. Chapter 8 presents a new theory of adult development that provides the foundation for a more comprehensive understanding of mature practice.

An Overview of the Mature Practice
Research Investigation

My study strongly suggests that a considerable number of experienced psychotherapy practitioners have limited confidence in the clinical procedures that they recommend to their patients. According to the first research investigation of the lives and clinical practices of highly experienced psychoanalysts and psychotherapists, a considerable number of those studied have had unsatisfactory personal therapy and are seriously disillusioned about the effectiveness of psychoanalysis and psychotherapy. When these practitioners were asked if they would consider "returning to the couch" in time of personal distress, these seasoned therapists stated categorically "no."

Do these mature practitioners have any more trust in their own analytic skills than in those of the colleagues from whom they refuse to request psychological help? Apparently not! The clinical training of the psychotherapist is built upon the belief that to the extent that the practitioner's self-examination is ignored, clinical competence will be compromised. Yet, when asked about their own self-examination, most of the experienced practitioners investigated reported that they use it infrequently because they have not developed any great skill with self-examination. Indeed, one very prominent psychiatrist referred to the process of self-analysis as "ridiculous." On the basis of these findings, it is not surprising that more than half of those studied characterized their clinical practice as having a detrimental effect on their relationships with family and significant others.

It is important to indicate that not all the senior practitioners involved in my study were pessimistic about their careers. Those practitioners I interviewed who were regarded by their colleagues as "master practitioners" were more vibrant and sanguine about their careers than most of the other senior practitioners. In the pages that follow I examine the life experiences and personality factors that appear to contribute to these master practitioners' ability to triumph over adversity and achieve maturity and wisdom in ways that many of their fellow senior colleagues have not.

The Vignettes

With the exception of George Valliant (1977), theorists of adult development have emphasized that mid-life for most people is a time of *existential crisis*. The vignettes that I present here examine issues in the lives and practices of senior practitioners that cause crises in their lives or in those of others with whom the practitioner is involved. From a storehouse of clinical material collected over the past twenty-five years I have chosen events in the lives of mature practitioners — some ubiquitous, some unusual, but all containing distinctive themes that touch upon the hopes, aspirations, vulnerabilities, and dissatisfactions common to most seasoned practitioners.

I have made changes in some of the stories to protect the identity of the participants and in still others to accentuate the critical issues involved in these events. Therefore, I offer these vignettes with a caution. I believe that the categories customarily used to characterize literature are quite misleading. Actually, literary works are never fictitious. Everything described in literature is purloined from life — viewed as the author needed to believe or would have liked the events to have occurred. The characters the author "invents" are people the author already knows and is seeking to come to terms with in a way he or she has not been able in the nonliterary world. Correspondingly, works of nonfiction are always "imagined." They represent the author's imago of the psychic reality of the people depicted. This reality is not limited by the facts actually known about the people being described, however, but rather by the dearth of creative inferences and tempered wisdom of the writer as to what is psychically existent in the characters.

In reading the accounts of therapists in conflict, the reader might well ask: "How are these conflicts specifically related to developmental issues of maturity rather than being issues that practitioners might become caught up in any time in their careers?"

Aging has a distinctive course of influence over our lives. Being a practitioner in mid-life and the years beyond offers us opportunities for an enlightened impact upon the lives of our patients and our colleagues. This wisdom comes both from our clinical experience and from having lived our own lives fully and well. Aging also has its dark side. We are exposed at mid-life to the hurts and vulnerabilities of heart and mind that were not issues — or at least not crucial concerns — in our younger days. No less importantly, the expectations at mid-life are also different from those in earlier seasons.

In Chapter 2 I discuss Alan, a psychiatrist who disdained desire. Alan's need for superiority was a direct response to his anxieties at age forty about his lack of creative accomplishment, as a psychoanalyst and in his music avocation. Marmor (1968), in one of the earliest articles on the crisis of middle age, pointed out that one of the major adjustments of mid-life for most people is facing the hard fact that the fantasized hopes of youth — for accomplishment, for wealth, and for romance — have not been achieved and have become improbable. When Alan faced the lack of time he had left to fulfill his desires, the defenses that had cloaked his deep despair could no longer work effectively. His desperate intrapsychic defensive structure at mid-life was mobilized to deny the reality of his own yearning.

At mid-life and beyond, many practitioners are placed in positions of responsibility for the future generation of practitioners. We expect senior practitioners to have had their expertise softened by the wisdom of their own life experiences, with an emphasis on compassion, decency, and common sense. As the story of the lonely psychiatrist in Chapter 2 shows, senior practitioners whose expert knowledge is based on the lives of others rather than on themselves can offer only limited perspectives about the human condition to their colleagues and patients.

AUDIENCE

This book is intended for the seasoned psychotherapist who is interested in reviewing and examining the issues that pertain to mature practice. It should be especially useful to the practitioner (seasoned or not) who is struggling with the dilemmas of clinical practice and would like some guidance as to whether his or her issues are developmental or more circumscribed to technical issues of clinical practice. This book also should be of interest to less experienced and neophyte therapists who wish to anticipate future issues in their careers. In this regard, it may serve as a significant text in the training programs of all psychotherapists and counselors so that these students may be better informed as to whether they are personally suited for the career of healer. Allen Wheelis (1956) has maintained that the vocation of psychotherapist misleads those who wish to pursue it as a career. According to Wheelis, psychotherapy is experienced quite differently by the practitioner than by the outsider. Psychotherapy, he claims, has certain qualities that cannot properly be put into words. They can only be found by experiencing them.

I am somewhat in disagreement with Wheelis. While it is true that many of the important processes of being a practitioner can only be realized by gradual steps and by exposure to one's own resources and vulnerabilities, I do believe that we can learn some very important lessons from other's experiences. This book is written from this ethos.

The Seasoned Psychotherapist explores the privilege of being a mature member of a select cadre of people who study the human psyche in the only way that it can be probed in-depth (Spuviell, 1984). And although psychotherapy can be a difficult and some times devastating responsibility, this book will show how the seasoned practitioner can use his tempered wisdom and maturity to live and practice fully and well. This book seeks to alert the practitioner to the personal and career issues that practitioners who have reached maturity have found influencing their lives. On the other hand, this is not a book about therapeutic technique. After all, information about technical issues is rarely the major concern of a senior practitioner. But changes in body, spirit, and social network are of vital interest and deeply influence his or her clinical work. Moreover, once any relatively psychologically healthy practitioner with adequate training comes to terms with his or her personal issues, technical considerations are relatively minor matters.

Finally, this book should be of interest to the general reader intrigued by psychology and personal growth and curious about what the experienced practitioners of the healing arts report about their own lives.

two

THE PSYCHIATRIST WHO
DISDAINED DESIRE

The most pressing existential crisis of our age is the pervasive sense of aloneness which so many of us feel so much of the time.

—G. V. Haigh, 1967

The wintering of age can be pitiless. Captive in lonely solitude, an aging analyst surrendered her capability to self-reflect. She became a divided soul, available to her patients in their analytic hours but no longer willing to respect her oath of confidentiality afterward.

When I lived in the south I became an acquaintance of Nora, an elderly, widowed psychiatrist who was regarded in psychiatric circles as the dean and chief spokesperson for the psychoanalytic community. Nora had been analyzed and trained by René Spitz, the eminent European theorist, researcher, and practitioner, who came to the United States in the 1930s.

When I met Nora, she had lost her husband a few years before and her children were living far away. In recent years she spent more time rescuing other people than living her own life. Her patients became her favorite topic of conversation. It was uncomfortable and embarrassing to hear intimate details about people I knew, including friends and supervisees, reported from their analytic sessions. In my presence and that of others, Nora discussed her patients by name, as if she was gossiping about neighbors. When it was suggested that her behavior was intriguing but wrong, she scoffed at the idea. She indicated that in her experience many renown analysts did the same.

Aging, with its ubiquitous accompaniment of loss of close and caring family and friends, may compound adverse tendencies practitioners are susceptible to throughout their careers. One of the most dangerous of these is *superiority* augmented by rigidity and encapsulation.

Let us be frank with each other. We as seasoned psychotherapists do not generally regard ourselves as ordinary people. We believe that in a number of particular ways we are exceptional. Generally, we believe that we are more intelligent, more compassionate, and more willing to express our perceptiveness about people in caring and concerned ways than are others. In some practitioners this constellation of beliefs may be more exaggerated than in others, resulting in what Ernest Jones referred to as "The God Complex." Jones suggested that many who are drawn to the healing professions have disavowed their own sense of impotence through an identification with the Supreme Being. People with this type of character structure evince intense scopophilia and curiosity about the private lives of others, together with a strong need to be recognized and admired for their superior skills in understanding and helping others understand themselves (Marmor, 1953).

A belief in their superiority has an ironic effect on the way that some senior practitioners view human behavior. It extols the observation of behavior while at the same time devaluing the direct experience of existence. We should not be surprised, then, that these practitioners regard themselves as experts on other people's behavior, while their patients are regarded as naive or deluded in understanding the intent of their own. Not recognizing that those who are aware only of their version of a situation know very little about that event, they fail to heed Goethe's caution that "Even superior talents will be obscured, defeated and destroyed if a man does not recognize the limits of his powers." Consequently, these practitioners act as if their psychological expertise unquestionably gave them the prerogative to steer patients away from what they purport to want and toward what they "actually need" in terms of their psychological development. In so doing they attempt to wrestle away the "illusion" of reality from the patient's idiosyncratic world view and to replace it with their own, "objective" reality.

The need to represent oneself with absolute certainty often results from attempts to deny a crisis in one's development. The following vignette examines the therapeutic actions that result from a practitioner's failure to appropriately respond to a long-standing developmental crisis in his life.

The prismed streaks of white light caught my eye as I sat in Dr. Sagemore's spacious Greenwich Village loft, with its twenty-foot ceiling and its numerous anterooms adjacent to this vast living room. My reconnaissance followed the light to a man I shall call "Alan," sitting cross-legged on a large, richly embroidered Pasha's Pillow. Alan is a small, bearded psychiatrist of indeterminate age, with sandy, thinning curls. His thick eyeglass lens were capturing the brilliant ray of winter sun, casting flashing arrows of light across the living room.

When Irving Sagemore left his psychoanalytic practice of thirty years, he gathered around him a group of former patients, colleagues, literary and artistic people. This group, who from their rhetoric and dress bore a sense of being mavericks, accompanied Irving on his yearly pilgrimage to visit and study with a renown Persian Sufi. One Sunday a month they held a salon among the worn and ill-matched furniture that conveyed bad memories of the Sagemores' previous marriages.

As I followed the streaks of refractured light to Alan, I wondered what I was doing in the midst of this curious twelve people. I had once respected Irving as an intellectual who led provocative workshops at psychoanalytic meetings I attended. I had heard that he had become disillusioned with being an analyst. Independently wealthy, he stopped practicing psychotherapy and stayed home to read books and write poetry. Clarissa Sagemore, his wife, is a professor of French literature, who was in her twelfth year of analysis at the time of this story. From her comments at the salon, I learned that she viewed psychoanalysis as a fascinating intellectual pursuit but had no idea that it was supposed to help people come to terms with their problems in living.

When I was given a reception for the publication of one of my books, I sent the Sagemores an invitation. Irving wrote back and suggested that, instead of their attending my reception, I join their salon. His letter mentioned that the Sunday afternoon salon was frequented by some highly creative and intellectual people, who were not bound by the strictures of conventional reality. I had hoped that in this setting I might find a band of kindred souls with whom to examine the personal concerns I had about the practice of psychotherapy and how it affected my life.

But once I heard Alan speak about his world view and noted the strong agreement of others in the room with his cynical rhetoric, I knew at once that I had come to the wrong place to broach my own personal concerns.

Alan informed us in his slow and very deliberate manner that "our human problem is that we desire and arduously strive for gratification that we can never have."

A gaunt older man, a graphic illustrator wrapped in a blanket with his feet up on the couch, asked Alan, "Just what is it that we all desire and cannot have?"

Alan removed his thick eyeglasses and carefully wiped them with a small blue silk handkerchief. "Desire," he informed us in a voice devoid of any discernible affect, "is a yearning to return to the gratifications that once were provided at the mother's breast. These satisfactions are no longer possible to obtain. Indeed, desire is a quest for a symbolic repetition of a pleasure whose attainment has become improbable."

I looked around the circle to see how the others were responding to Alan's disconcerting view of the human condition. Several seemed puzzled. But not the Sagemores. They were beaming proudly. "Continue!" urged Irving enthusiastically.

Alan smiled faintly and informed us in his carefully chosen words, "Since we have no control over what happens to us, striving, planning and cooperating with other people have no real effect on our actual fate. The best that we can do is not to complain or even to struggle and fight. Instead, we must relinquish our desires without regret or, indeed, any other emotion. This is because there is no such thing as a constructive emotion. Genuine love may be occasionally exhibited by an adult towards a child, but genuine feeling is rarely evinced between adults. So-called 'positive' emotions are nothing more than ineffectual, passive, and magically hoped-for ways of pliantly waiting for change to happen in one's life."

Alan's stoic attitude disturbed me. It may well serve his own illusions to believe as he did, but he professed to be a psychotherapist, not an academic philosopher. How does he respond to his patients' attempts to secure his assistance, I wondered, if he really believes that none of us can be of help to anyone else? I pointedly asked him about this.

Alan did not look in my direction as I questioned him, as though he did not wish to acknowledge my question, or me. Instead, he again removed his glasses and carefully wiped them. He slowly moni-

tored the faces in the circle. As he looked at other people, his perpet-
ually partially opened mouth conveyed a countenance of continual
sarcasm.

"I submit," sharply asserted Clarissa Sagemore, as if on cue, "what
Alan does in his private office is none of our business. Why should he
have to tell us anything about it?"

"Oh, do tell us what you do with patients when you close your
door!" exclaimed the man in the blanket, with a mischievous giggle.
Alan ignored him. He looked at Clarissa as if he might accept her
gesture of immunity. But then something changed in Alan's expression. With a tilt of his head he addressed my question, "I'll tell you
precisely what I do in my clinical practice. My job consists only of
enabling my patients to realize that they cannot depend on me or, by
implication, anyone else for their salvation. When they finally realize
this, they don't have to return to see me, because they are fully
capable of living without intention or desire. Only then can they fully
appreciate what is and what is not possible for them."

To me Alan's account of his practice sounded as abstract and
vague as it seemed absurd. Did he really mean what he seemed to be
saying about successful treatment consisting of discouraging the patient from caring and cooperative efforts with other people? I wondered. I asked him for a clinical illustration.

"Recently, I have been seeing in treatment an insufferably dependent woman," he reported. "My treatment of her problem consists of
telling her as she enters my office every week to 'put the $125 on the
table and leave the office promptly.' If she lingers in the office I turn
my chair away from where she is standing and read a book or something like that. Of course, I say 'good-bye' as she walks out the door.
She has not returned and I have not heard from her in the last three or
four weeks."

Was Alan's account factual? I do not know. But I do believe that it
was a serious response to my asking him to present the implications
of his world view in his therapeutic practice.

Is Alan a maverick practitioner, whose lack of professional qualifi-
cations renders his situation of little implication for the well-trained,
experienced practitioner for whom I am writing? Alan completed a
conventional psychiatric residency program and has a certificate
from a respected psychoanalytic training institute. He also was a
patient and later a supervisee of Irving Sagemore.

Despite seasoned practitioners' extraordinary preparation for examining the human psyche, they share with everyone else the frailties

of being merely human in an imperfect world, as the results of the research investigation reported in later chapters sometimes painfully demonstrates. To understand Alan's therapeutic practice, we need to examine his psychological struggles from the perspective of his own subjectivity.

Alan's frailties were involved with a sense of the tragic in regard to his creative talents with which he had never come to terms. Earlier in his life his ambition was to be a serious classical music composer. Even though he has had several of his sonatas played by major orchestras, he has never been able to regard himself as a serious composer. He explained this contradiction by claiming that *real* musicians are able to support themselves with their creative efforts and to spend most of their time being artists rather than in some other profession. Alan's musical projects had not been in sufficient demand to be financially successful.

His artistic ambition was enmeshed in his relationship with his father. His father came from a musical family but had to abandon a musical career in coming to the United States from Europe, in order to support his family.

As long as Alan could remember, his parents worked six or more days a week at the most difficult and unsatisfying types of labor. It was their priority, nevertheless, that Alan and his sister go to a distant school, world famous for its music program.

When he was a child, Alan experienced being taken with his sister to the railroad station for the long trip back to school after a holiday at home as painful. The sadness he felt at those moments was not anticipated homesickness. He actually preferred to be in the happy atmosphere of his school than with his hard-to-please parents. Sitting in the train at the station with one of his parents waiting outside, he could never for longer than a moment focus on the face he saw through the window of the train. The face would always be worn and tired. Though it showed a smile of reassurance, he did not feel comforted. He felt too ashamed of being sent to a school for which his parents were so valiantly struggling to pay.

He experienced similar discomfort when home from school on holidays. When asked how he spent that day, or worse, when "caught" in his room writing a short story or a poem, Alan felt considerable humiliation. His father regarded these pursuits as trivial and self-serving, considering how he worked at real jobs to support his family. Musical ambitions his father could understand and, of course, studies that would train Alan for a profession in which he could make a good livelihood. But all the writers he knew of were starving. "The more education you get," his father told him more than once, "the dumber you seem to be."

Alan tried to compensate for his self-doubts by becoming a diligent student. He gained considerable recognition for his intellect from teachers and classmates. He earned excellent scholarships to both college and medical school. After finishing medical school, he entered a psychiatric residency training program and then completed analytic training. He found that he had no difficulty understanding the plights of his patients. He was well-trained and carried out the analyses just as he had been taught.

But something was lacking: he would not allow his patients to affect him deeply. His coldness, as other perceived it, concerned him painfully during his training and early into his career. But his first personal analysis during his residency did him little good, aside from uncovering the source of his self-contempt as his attempts to please his demanding father and gain his approval and pride. His analyst, Alan believed, was emotionally and intellectually impeded by the institutional conventions of his analytic doctrine, so that he categorically reduced all questions of suffering in a person's life to issues of unresolved oedipal guilt. Alan did not believe that he was harboring any considerable degree of conscious or unconscious guilt. He certainly did not feel that he hated or was competing with the old man. Whatever he really felt, he believed that it included admiration for the man in the way he had been willing to work for what he held to be important. Yet working hard didn't seem to be the answer for Alan. It seemed too magically involved with an assumed rational universe that rewarded people fairly for their good intentions and efforts.

Early in his therapeutic career his confusion as to how best to make some sense of the human condition was continually being examined in light of the psychological tools he was acquiring clinically each day. It seemed to him that the ways that his patients came to terms with their suffering consisted of shallow and self-deluding rationalizations. These ploys at feeling better with oneself were intellectually unacceptable to Alan.

Alan realized that the longer he practiced psychotherapy the more his ways of responding to his patients were being informed by his despair. But when one has been hurt for as long as he had been, these bruised feelings finally become acceptable and almost comfortable, like worn old leather. One day Alan could no longer remember feeling dissatisfied with his coldness and cynicism toward his patients.

Since it is rare for two practitioners to agree on a clinical matter, the tools are readily available to the intellectually astute practitioner for bolstering his self-delusion about the soundness of his clinical work. The meaningfulness of the life of the practitioner who is in despair does not wane categorically. It departs from his confidence and sense of well-being bit by bit (Wheelis, 1962). Therefore, through the tricks of the trade the seasoned practitioner may still carry out his professional duties almost competently, even when his convictions about the unsoundness of his theory and the illusory benefits of his clinical work should be evident to him (Goldberg, 1991).

By the time Alan had become a seasoned practitioner he could no longer recognize his despair and the doubts that he had once harbored about his clinical work. To have done so would have compelled Alan to acknowledge that he had a serious emotional disturbance. Because he had never been able to resolve for himself his pervasive and crippling sense of shame and unworthiness, Alan sought to escape from his anguish by denying it and rationalizing that his cynicism was preferable to naive desires in human affairs.

Alan's denial was destructively abetted by his analytic role, which allowed him to be fascinated by the psychopathology of his patients. His denial was ironic, in that his suffering caused him to deny his commonality with his patients and instead to assume a superiority over the "shallow" and "self-deluded" people he encountered in the world. Because of his "identification denial," he did not feel very involved with his patients and didn't really know them too well. Nor, of course, would he permit them to get close to him. Some of his patients had picked up that he was distressed. In these situations, Alan used his analytic role to remain distant. He focused on his patients' attempts to express concern for him as, if not exactly inappropriate, then certainly manipulative and insincere. In order to protect himself from the awareness that his patients might be solicitous toward him because he was hurt and suffering, he viewed their attempts at caring for him as not genuinely motivated, but as disguised efforts to please some significant person in their past whom Alan psychologically represented.

Just as one of the inner driving forces that compelled some of Alan's classmates in medical school to become pathologists was their unrecognized fear of their helplessness in the face of their own mortality, a major compelling and unwitting force in Alan's becoming a psychoanalyst was the opportunity to learn sophisticated ways of denying that he was a person who was subject to the same fears and trepidations as "ordinary people." In the face of his helplessness in trying to understand his demanding and seemingly never pleased parents, who induced so much shame in him for what they had given him, Alan as a child had not developed a personal identity that gave him a sense of security and feelings of well-being. He used that personal attribute which had been the most admired by others to forge a good feeling about himself. This is to say, using his intellect, he found a fund of knowledge and a method of inquiry into human affairs that set him apart from others in dealing with the human condition.

We may well wonder why Alan's intellect and clinical training did not function critically as well as defensively and force him to recognize that he was not promoting his patients' psychological growth, that he was, in fact, being destructive to them. Unfortunately, Alan went into his training analysis and later continued as a supervisee and devoted disciple of Irving Sagemore. Despite his ostensible charm, generosity, and liberalness, Irving is a hard-bitten cynic. It was Irving who encouraged Alan's "no desire" world view. Indeed, it was Irving's disdaining attitude, couched in his helping gestures, that had drawn Alan to Irving for analysis. Irving had given a presentation on the creative process in poetry to the local psychoanalytic institute society at which he was a prominent training analyst. Alan was so impressed with Irving's intellect that he went up to him at the end of the lecture and told him that he was a beginning candidate at the institute and that he had published some poems while a college undergraduate. Irving enthusiastically asked him to send him copies of his best poems. Within a week Alan received the poems back. They had been very carefully read. Indeed, almost every word had either been crossed out or changed. Irving had entirely rewritten Alan's poems as Irving apparently believed they should have been written originally. There was something about Irving's unshakable self-righteousness that had deeply impressed Alan and brought him under Irving's aegis.

Alan is a type of practitioner virtually ignored in the clinical literature. I call practitioners like Alan "as if" therapists. They are people who have experienced considerable psychic conflict in their lives before becoming therapists. They regard their personal analysis or therapy as having saved their lives. With gratitude to their therapists for their survival, they decide to dedicate their lives to providing help for troubled people in much the same way that their therapists did for them. If they are fortunate they may find a senior practitioner who will resist getting embroiled with them in therapy suffused with highly charged transference and countertransference issues. A skilled therapist will not fall prey to these patients' attempts to manipulate the therapist into making direct interventions in the patients' lives and by so doing becoming a significant substratum of the patients' social and emotional life.

If these individuals get involved with highly narcissistic and charismatic therapists like Irving, on the other hand, the relationship will become more than a therapeutic and professional one. It will consist of an enmeshed mentorship in which the cast of characters for each becomes thoroughly confused. In this unfortunate situation, personal therapy will not resolve pervasive feelings of shame and unworthiness. Instead, becoming a psychotherapist serves for these "as if" practitioners as an inappropriate "strategy" for trying to disguise and deny their serious psychopathology. In perceiving a sense of shame in other people similar to them that they themselves harbor, they feel appalled by their own desperation, dependency, and failure to secure meaningful intimacy. In trying to deny this hateful image of themselves, they feel compelled to act superior to others, especially their patients. They try to secure their patients' admiration for them so that their patients will feel about them the same way as they did about their own personal analysts or therapists.

I relate Alan's story not because I believe that his character structure is representative of most seasoned practitioners, but because it illustrates the forces in our profession that serve to insulate practitioners from critically examining their clinical practices and world views. These are practices for which they and their patients pay a terrible price. These practices also poison the well for all of us who need the public trust in our position of healer.

The issues of clinical practice are different at mid-life and the years beyond than when practitioners start their psychotherapeutic career in their twenties or thirties. Alan's need for superiority was accentuated at mid-life, because this is typically the time at which one assesses one's life accomplishments. Alan's defensive structure at age forty was mobilized to avert his despair in not having achieved his life ambitions. He especially needed at this time in his life to deny the importance of desire. In the next chapter I will discuss what experienced practitioners have written about their own personal experiences with maturity, as reported in the psychoanalytic and psychological literature.

three

THE PERILS OF BEING
A SEASONED PRACTITIONER

Oh damned despair, to shun the living light and plunge
thy shameful soul in endless night!

—Lucretius, *De Rerum Nature*

What do we know about the old masters of psychoanalysis and
psychotherapy that can help us with the way we practice and conduct
our lives as senior practitioners today? An extensive search of the
psychoanalytic and psychological literature reveals that the master
practitioners who came before us, although leaving us with a rich
legacy of theory and technique, have written very little about the
personal effect of their middle and senior years on their practices.

Three of the most prominent practitioners of the past—Freud,
Jung, and Rogers—seemed to have increasingly lost interest in conducting psychotherapy when they reached senior maturity. They
spent more of their time than in their younger days writing theoretical papers and applying what they had learned from their clinical
experiences to broad social issues. Freud (1935) tells us in the post-
script to his autobiography of the regressive development of his last
contributions to psychoanalysis:

But I myself find that a significant change has come about.
Threads which in the course of my development had become
intertangled have now begun to separate; interests which I had

acquired in the later part of my life have receded, while the older and original ones become prominent once more. (p. 71).

Freud also appeared to have been rather disheartened by what he regarded as the lack of importance of his later work. He indicates that after 1923,

I have made no further decisive contributions to psycho-analy-sis: what I have written on the subject since then has been either unessential or would soon have been supplied by someone else. (p. 72)

The physical fatigue of aging may be a factor that wears down practitioners as they mature and contributes to the older practition-er's despair in finding meaning in the sunset of their lives. In her biography notes about Jung (1989), Jaffe wrote of his last years:

No bounds could ever be set willingly to his questioning and inquiring spirit, but his body was tired, too tired to stand up to the demands of another round of creative work. (p. 115)

Carl Rogers (1975) also wrote of the physical strain of aging in reporting on his forty-six years as a practitioner:

I am no longer actively engaged in individual therapy or empiri-cal research. (I am finding out as one passes seventy, there are physical limitations on what one can do.) (p. 143)

Physical health alone, however, does not explain the changes in the master practitioner's activities and interests. Jaffe indicated that she found in preparing with Jung his autobiography that

During the years in which the book was taking shape a process of transformation was also taking place in Jung. With each succeeding chapter he moved, as it were, farther away from himself, until at last he was able to see himself as well as the significance of his life and work from a distance. (Jung, 1989, p. vii)

To Jaffe's perspective Rogers (1975) added that, while his whole approach to people and their relationships changed only slowly as he aged, his understanding of how to apply his values and beliefs were recast markedly. Similar to Freud and Jung, he became interested in the ways that the educational principles of his therapeutic system could expand its reach beyond individuals and be taught to many more people through a well conceived educational program.

All three of these master practitioners expressed considerable disappointment in how few of their own cherished ideas were well received by their colleagues at the time of their conception. They also expressed reluctance in openly discussing these disappointments. For example, Freud (1935) breaks off and ends his autobiography by indicating that the public has no right to learn more of his personal struggles and disappointments than he had openly and frankly written about earlier in his career. This is understandable in that Freud felt that the revelation of his own self-examination found in his original writings had not been well treated by many of his colleagues. He cautioned others not to follow his example. Jung (1989) took a more historical and universal perspective on the reception of his work in his lifetime:

> If I ask the value of my life, I can only measure myself against the centuries and then I say, "Yes, it means something. Measured by the ideas of today, it means nothing." (p. xii)

The disappointment of Freud, Jung, and Rogers at the time of their contributions is somewhat understandable. They were highly innovative and creative theorists, as well as longtime practitioners. It is an unfortunate but frequent occurrence that highly creative thinkers are misunderstood and underappreciated in their lifetimes. But what of less exceptional senior practitioners?

There are numerous studies of the satisfactions and disappointments in the careers of younger practitioners (for example, Farber and Heifetz, 1981, 1982; Henry, Sims, and Spray, 1971, 1973); however, there is only one empirical study that evaluates the issues and concerns of the senior practitioner. Kelly and his associates' (1978) long-term follow-up study of those who started their careers as clinical psychology trainees at Veterans Administration hospitals found that a strong disappointment in the career of being a psychology practitioner was a pervasive attitude among these psychologists. In Kelly et al.'s study, clinical psychology interns assessed in 1947 were surveyed as practitioners of a decade in 1957 and as senior practitioners twenty-five years after their internship. For the group, scholarly production was minimal. Satisfaction with their choice of career, which was low at the ten-year mark, was even lower at twenty-five. Therapists and researchers were the least satisfied. Among this group of psychologists, diagnosticians and teachers reported that they were the most content in their careers.

We have seen that the master practitioners of the past have reported little on the issues of mature practice. Have senior practitioners in recent times provided more pertinent information? Hardly! The only study I found that empirically examines the clinical work of experienced practitioners was one in which Whitehorn (1960) demonstrated that at different ages psychiatrists with different personality structures relate differently to patients. Some of these age-related therapeutic styles click better with some patients than they do with others. It would appear that not every patient in Whitehorn's study related best to the most experienced therapist.

Even impressionistic reports on mature practice are difficult to find. Those that are in the literature are usually concerned with the influence of illness on the aging practitioner. Weiner (1990) found in his interviews with fifteen older psychiatrists that they, like other older people deeply involved in their work, continue to practice as long as they possibly can and cite poor health as the main reason for their retirement. In a recent article entitled, "Wounded Healers," Maeder (1989) maintained that many psychotherapists seem unwilling to leave their practices when they have reached retirement age because of their need to be needed. Dewald (1981), in discussing the impact of personal illness on mature practice, suggests that countertransferential narcissism is involved in much of the adverse effect of illness in the aging practitioner. The anxiety and conflict aroused by personal illness, Dewald reports, is generally handled by denial, as the therapist enacts the wish to avoid taking the topic seriously. Eissler (1977) gives some support to Dewald's view. He found that the analyst's narcissistic involvement in patients' material heightens in the older analyst; however, Eissler indicates that there are some positive consequences of the aged analyst's narcissism, in addition to its many problems (see Chapter 7).

The only book on aspects of mature practice was a book edited by Arthur Burton (1972) that provided autobiographic accounts of twelve prominent psychotherapists' lives. Since these stories covered their entire careers and were written while each was still practicing, only limited aspects of senior practice were described.

THE PERILS OF MATURE PRACTICE

I am sitting in my office at 7:00 AM, waiting for my first patient of the day, as I review the literature on mature practice in the context of my own clinical mind-set. As I canvass the welter of clinical situations that I have either personally experienced or been told of, I recognize that a serious omission in the literature on psychotherapeutic practice is a frank discussion of how the fantasy of youthful practice contrasts with the realities of being a mature psychotherapist.

One of the central sources of disillusionment for mature practitioners has to do with their fantasy as beginners of the skillful ease of practice as one becomes "seasoned." As beginners, they expected their clinical endeavors to be difficult, unsure, and often unsuccessful. But few anticipated that after years of experience it would continue to be difficult. The assumption was that with maturity psychotherapeutic practice would become easy and comfortable, like a well-practiced tennis stroke. The young practitioner's fantasy foretold a ceaseless volley of wise and healing interpretations, launched with elegance, ease, and accuracy.

The seasoned practitioner experiences the therapeutic endeavor quite differently from what was imagined as a neophyte. The work is still arduous. Psychotherapy for the experienced practitioner, as for the beginner, continues to have its uncertainties and failures. Psychotherapy is not a science that can be decisively mastered. It continues to be difficult because there is never a final and perfect therapy form that can be endlessly manufactured for all diverse clinical situations and individuals.

At its best psychotherapy is a courageous and compassionate healing craft. We must come to unique terms with each patient who enters our consulting room. Even as seasoned practitioners we may have to struggle painfully with personal issues that we had assumed were long ago resolved. One of the most important of these is feeling *inspired* in our work. In this regard I am reminded of a practitioner whom I will call "Norman Ross." Norman had been an important supervisor and mentor during my early career. I felt appreciative toward him for his encouraging me to develop creative ways to work analytically with patients while I was in training.

Ten years later, soon after I left my marriage, I attended a psychotherapy conference in New Orleans. During the conference I met both Norman and an attractive woman psychologist. My former supervisor, who recently had terminated a long-term marriage, seemed lonely and I encouraged him to join us on a boat trip up the Mississippi River and on other excursions we took during our stay in New Orleans. After a while I became aware of being annoyed about Norman's accompanying us, although I wasn't sure why. I had always found Norman to be lively and witty. On the third day, my female friend said to me, "I think that you have outgrown your former supervisor. He keeps trying to pull you back to when he was supervising you at the beginning of your career." I realized then that my annoyance with Norman was with his implicitly demanding that I be in a place where I no longer wished or needed to be.

Aging is difficult for most people. What enables us to tolerate the losses of growing older is the wisdom maturity offers us about how to live with more inspiration than we had when we were younger. This inspiration enables us to stay vibrant. Aging without wisdom leads to intense despair about what we have lost and for which we have not been compensated.

Some practitioners are able to stay wise and inspired throughout their careers by their uncanny skill of finding new mentors for themselves when they outlive or outgrow their teachers. Robert Butler, the eminent gerontologist and psychiatrist, I was told by his wife, has been able all of his life to find a person older than himself, even when he was past sixty, to serve as a mentor and guide.

Sometimes mentors serve us best not by the continuing of their relationship with us, but by wisely alerting us about where to find inspiration for living and practicing fully and well.

Shortly after my disappointing meeting with Norman Ross in New Orleans, I was invited to conduct a workshop on group psychotherapy skills to a cadre of skeptical veteran psychiatrists who lived in isolated communities in Alaska. Honored to be requested to fly across the continent at a very generous professional fee, I tried to reach these seasoned practitioners with a dazzling display of interpersonal techniques. They were not impressed. Finally, one of the most senior of this group said to me in a subdued voice, "Relax, we're not in a hurry! We have all left the haste and madness of the lower forty-eight states because we are in no hurry to find something. Besides, the answers to our questions are all around us if we are quiet awhile and open to the answers that our questions bring us."

In the chapters to follow I will present the responses that 64 highly experienced practitioners offered to me about where to look and how best to use being a mature examiner of the human psyche to live a wise and authentic life.

— four —

THE BASIC ASSUMPTIONS OF THE MATURE PRACTICE RESEARCH PROJECT

The world is but a school of inquiry.

—Montaigne, *Essays*

Because no empirical data had been published with regard to the crucial issues in the personal lives and professional practices of experienced psychotherapists, I decided to collect this information myself. My overall research interest was embedded in the question: *"What do seasoned practitioners do in their work and how do they feel about themselves and their patients that differ from when they were beginners?"*

To answer my research question, I adopted five investigatory strategies:

1. I included in my research sample members of the four prominent mental health disciplines—psychoanalysis, psychiatry, psychology and social work.
2. For potential respondents to my research investigation, I sought out practitioners from throughout the United States and Canada.
3. I tried to include representatives from diverse cultural and ethnic groups. Previous investigators (Burton, 1972; Henry et al., 1971) had concluded that their findings were representative of a

highly circumscribed ethnic-cultural grouping, rather than reflecting the lives and sentiments of psychotherapists across cultures.

4. I decided that the most fecund and efficient method for me to collect information about how self-examined and highly articulate people conduct their lives was a combination of questionnaires and in-depth personal interviews.

5. In order to evaluate my findings in the context of what is already empirically known about the personal concerns of psychotherapists, I compared the findings of my study with the two empirical studies previously conducted with regard to aspects of psychotherapeutic practice that are experienced as satisfying or stressful (Farber and Heifetz, 1981, 1982).

Despite following these research strategies, I can make no claim that my findings are representative of the entire senior psychotherapist population in the United States or anywhere else. The findings of my study are limited by several factors. Questionnaires that probe people's private lives, no matter how well formulated, generally do not have high rates of returns. This is one of the reasons why surveys are sent out in large numbers. In planning my study I was faced with a major consideration. Because my funds for carrying out this study were limited, I needed to ensure the largest possible return of completed questionnaires relative to the number I sent out. Mailing questionnaires to a randomly selected group of senior practitioners was not cost efficient. I had another option. I assumed that I would get a considerably higher return of completed questionnaires from practitioners who knew me personally and believed that I would not misuse the information they sent me. Therefore, in this exploratory research project, I decided to sacrifice some representativeness of my sample of informants by sending the questionnaires to seasoned practitioners whom I knew personally or whose professional reputation was such that I believed that their interest in research would likely stimulate their cooperation.

The study was also limited by a self-selection process inherent in voluntarily filling out and returning the information. A large number of practitioners did not return the questionnaires sent them. I mailed 200 questionnaires and received 52 completed.

In short, I do not tacitly assume that my research findings are representative of experienced psychotherapists of all the different theoretical persuasions or from every corner of the world. There is a disproportionate representation of seasoned practitioners who are oriented toward theoretical formulations that are psychoanalytic, psychodynamic, existential, or humanistic. Generally, these are the practitioners with whom I have the closest personal associations. Behavioral or cognitive psychotherapists may live and practice their profession differently from my respondents. Furthermore, the information collected is representative primarily of conditions in the United States and Canada.

On the other hand, it is quite possible that my data do capture the concerns of most seasoned practitioners. There is something about being a healer, regardless of the precise way that one's clinical practice is formulated, that draws us together as practitioners and suggests that we probably have some crucial core values in common. This is more likely to be true of experienced practitioners with different theoretical points of view than of beginners. The empirical research of Fred Fiedler (1950) tends to verify this contention. He has shown that as therapists become more experienced their work tends to be more similar to that of other senior therapists of different theoretical orientations than to that of less experienced therapists of their own persuasion.

THEORETICAL ASSUMPTIONS

The questionnaire (which is found in the Appendix) was designed to provide information about mature practice based on the following assumptions:

I assumed that there are important issues and concerns that practitioners encounter in their mature years of practice that they didn't anticipate when they started their careers. Carl Rogers (1975) indicated that when he looked back over nearly fifty years of practice "the major element of my reaction was surprise" at what the work consisted of and how it was received by one's colleagues. The significant issues of psychotherapeutic practice, when recognized, can be of critical value to all practitioners, not just experienced ones. Wheelis (1956) lamented that it is usually at mid-career that practitioners decide that their career was chosen for the wrong reasons. At that point they believe it is too late to do much about their commitment of two or three decades past. Obviously, the health of our profession and that of its practitioners would be better served if students and beginners had some reliable information upon entering the portals of their career to guide them in whether or not they are embarking on the right path.

I was interested in the ways that the practitioners' views about neurosis and human nature had changed over the years of practice. I assumed that one of the most important factors to investigate was whether there had been any significant change in how the practitioner now regarded and responded to human suffering. I also assumed that, whatever the practitioner's own source of personal suffering had been, this angst would be significant in understanding current functioning as a psychotherapist. It is probably safe to say that practitioners who are floundering in their clinical work are adrift in their private lives as well. Therefore, I planned to query practitioners about how their life issues had decisively modified their youthful values. Many neophyte therapists, I have found from my experience as a psychotherapy educator, view psychoanalysis and psychotherapy as finely attuned rational tools that can successfully resolve all types of emotional conflict. Many of them seem to believe that the art and science of psychotherapy can be steadily mastered with clinical experience and perseverance, regardless of one's own painful internal struggles. After many years of clinical experience, including periods of disillusionment, I have a less fervent faith in psychological insight and my own expertise, having replaced this faith with more trust in my patients' inner wisdom and the healing capacities of compassion, decency, and common sense. I was curious about the extent to which other experienced practitioners shared these observations.

I also was curious about the lessons that seasoned practitioners had learned from their patients. Those who are called to the profession of psychological healer generally pursue it with an intense interest in finding out about themselves. They have found a career that provides them with a continuous means for examining their own lives. I inquired about the seasoned practitioners' personal analysis or psychotherapy as well as their self-examination (self-analysis). I assumed that, unless practitioners continue to examine their own lives after completing their apprenticeship, they will feel restive and bored. Practitioners who are still available for further personal growth, I further assumed, will be curious about the inner happenings of their patients in terms of what they can learn about themselves.

A well-known line from a poem by William Butler Yeats tells us that "a man must choose perfection of the life, or the work." Yeats was referring specifically to the life of the creative person. I was

curious whether his statement held true for therapists as well as artists. I assumed that creative wisdom derives at least as much from the
practitioner's private life as from his or her clinical practice. Therefore, to reiterate, I expected that those who were experiencing distress
in their professional practice would also be experiencing disappointments in their private life. I anticipated that the sources for both
disappointment and satisfaction in practice could be tapped by asking practitioners about their personal myth. In my experience, each
of us has a prototypic story about him- or herself that has direct
implications for how that person regards the world—its resources,
opportunities, and impediments to the achievement of that person's
desires.

For two major reasons I confined myself to only certain questions
and not to many other important concerns for the seasoned practitioner. First, to reasonably expect more than a few completed questionnaires, I needed to condense my investigation to a small number
of questions. Second, when I originally designed the study, I simply
wasn't aware of some of the important information I could have
sought from responses to the questionnaire. As I will discuss in
Chapter 7, I used the face-to-face interviews, which were conducted
for the most part after collecting the data from the questionnaires, to
gather information I didn't get from the questionnaires.

— five —

FIFTY-TWO EXPERIENCED PSYCHOTHERAPISTS EXAMINE THEIR CAREERS

> Like literary men, psychologists too speak of other men's emotions. But what of their passions. . . . A description of someone else's emotion is one thing. And our problem is to understand, for *me (us)* subjectively, what it is *to have* an emotion.
>
> — Robert Solomon, *The Passions*

The fifty-two seasoned psychotherapists — 37 men and 15 women — who discuss their careers in this chapter are a highly experienced group. They have a mean average of 30.35 years of clinical experience. Two of the psychiatrists have been practitioners for more than a half century. Of the forty-eight who practice full-time, their mean average years of full-time practice is 26.82. Further information on the background of these fifty-two practitioners follows:

Profession

Number of Psychologists	33	Number of social workers	4
Number of Psychiatrists	15		

Gender

Number of men	37	Number of women	15

Nationality

U.S.A.	47	Switzerland	1
Canada	4		

Theoretical Orientation

Psychoanalytic	9	Symbolic Experiential	1
Psychodynamic	9	Modern Psychoanalytic	1
Existential-Humanistic	5	Cognitive Psychoanalytic	1
Sullivanian	5	Horneyian	1
Object Relations	4	Bowen Family Systems	1
Self Psychology	3	Crisis Mobilization	1
Eclectic	3	Transactional Analysis	1
Systems Theory	2	Gestalt	1
Ego Psychology	1	Psychosynthesis	1
(Erik) Eriksonian	1	No designation	1

The first question on the questionnaire was:

As a seasoned practitioner, please list what have been the significant issues, concerns and dilemmas that you have encountered in practice that you did not anticipate before entering the career of psychotherapist (perhaps not even as a beginner).

Tables 1 and 2 list the categories of significant concern for the respondents. They differentiate these issues in terms of gender and professional discipline. The total number of responses exceed the number of respondents, as most respondents cited more than one significant concern.

For most of the respondents being a psychotherapist is like being in the Marines — it is a constant struggle. On the other hand, most of them reported that they had gained over the years a deeper understanding of and appreciation for the *complexity* of the human mind. Still others indicated that they had become disillusioned by the nature of the work. They stated that they had not earlier in their careers recognized how difficult it is to change people. Most of these seasoned practitioners seem to be still searching for a *guiding perspective*, a way of understanding their patients and themselves that would be more accurate and enlightening than what they realize now was the "misguided" theories that they had been taught as novices or had happened upon earlier in their careers. Through the years they have found these theories to be deficient. Typical in this regard is the statement from a psychiatrist with three decades of clinical experience:

TABLE 1: Significant Concerns

Concern	Males (37)		Females (15)		Total	
	n	%	n	%	n	%
Financial issues and working conditions	19	51.4	4	26.7	23	44.2
Clinical stress in working with patients	10	27.0	5	33.3	15	28.8
Legal concerns and professional politics	8	21.6	5	33.3	13	25
Countertransference	10	27.0	3	20	13	25
Ethical and moral issues	8	21.6	2	13.3	10	19.2
Theoretical limitations of their training	6	16.2	0	0	6	11.5
Isolation in practice	3	8.1	1	6.7	4	7.7
Adversive effects on family and other significant personal relationships	2	5.4	1	6.7	3	5.8
Self-esteem tied to therapeutic success	2	5.4	0	0	2	3.8
Retirement issues	2	5.4	0	0	2	3.8
Need for colleagial support	0	0	1	6.7	1	1.9
Difficulties terminating with patients	1	2.7	0	0	1	1.9
Invasion of Personhood	1	2.7	0	0	1	1.9

When I trained, psychotherapy was supposed to greatly ameliorate the so-called psychosomatic disorders, including peptic ulcer, high blood pressure and obesity. It took a few years of practice to find out that it didn't, and in fact often made these patients less comfortable. It also took a few years to realize that insight-oriented psychotherapy is not widely applicable and that the rapid development of a transference neurosis pointed more to severe ego impairment than to a successful outcome of therapy.

The practitioners' responses to subsequent questions suggested that a number of those queried believe that they have already found or will eventually find an enlightened perspective on what the human condition is all about. They now recognize, in a way they had not as beginners, that their enlightenment as practitioners comes not so much from what they learn clinically about patients as from the extensive work on themselves that is required in order to respond fully

TABLE 2: Significant Concerns by Profession

Concern	Psychi- atrists (15)		Psychol- ogists (33)		Social Workers (4)	
	n	%	n	%	n	%
Financial issues and working conditions	6	40	15	45.5	2	50
Clinical stress in working with patients	4	26.7	10	30.3	3	75
Legal concerns and professional politics	4	26.7	9	27.3	0	0
Countertransference	3	20	9	27.3	1	25
Ethical and moral issues	5	33.3	5	15.2	0	0
Theoretical limitations of their training	3	20	3	9.1	0	0
Isolation in practice	1	6.7	2	6.1	1	25
Adversive effects on family and other significant personal relationships	2	13.3	0	0	1	25
Self-esteem tied to therapeutic success	0	0	2	6.1	0	0
Retirement issues	0	0	2	6.1	0	0
Need for colleagial support	0	0	1	3.0	0	0
Difficulties terminating with patients	1		0	0	0	0
Invasion of personhood	1		0	0	0	0

to the exquisite nuances of the human condition they share with their patients during therapeutic dialogue. This is particularly critical in dealing with their anxiety with regard to their responsibilities toward people who are suffering.

Several respondents emphasized that psychotherapy works best when it is recognized as requiring the same ingredients as other good relationships. Still other practitioners qualified this point of view by indicating that a therapeutic relationship cannot reasonably be regarded as simply another relationship, since there are special demands on the therapist that are usually not present in informal relationships. Said differently, there was some difference of opinion as to whether a friendship model or a more traditional doctor-patient arrangement was the most appropriate and efficacious for therapeutic work. The practitioners who emphasized the former stressed the need for authentic caring in competent psychotherapy. The latter group tended to emphasize the need for careful diagnostic assessment, particularly in order to recognize early in the work that one is treating a "borderline" personality who requires special considerations, including the need to protect oneself from invasion into one's selfhood. Practitioners who expressed these cautions also were those who were concerned with the political struggles among practitioners and with the influence of institutional policies, such as those that involve health insurance, on clinical practice. In addition, they tended to be among those who pointed to the unpleasantness of the business aspects of practice, stressing the long hours and the need to work continually on getting referrals.

Several practitioners pointed out that there have been radical changes in the mental health field in the last couple of decades. From criticism within the field, as well as from outside, the general public has come to recognize that standard psychotherapeutic services — and especially psychoanalysis — are not the panacea they were touted to be for decades. More than ever before those looking around for psychological services are demanding short-term, symptom-specific treatment, rather than open-ended character reconstruction. In the past, seasoned practitioners could usually maintain as large a private practice as they liked, because most referrals sought or expected long-term treatment. Today, senior practitioners, who for many years have had full practices, are scurrying around trying to find referrals instead of having a waiting list of patients.

Moreover, in the past clinical experience was more venerated than it is today; consequently, working with a senior practitioner was usually preferable to therapy with a younger one. Today, innovative technological developments have modified societal attitudes about experience. The newer schools of psychotherapy offer short-term, highly specific modalities that place many highly experienced but traditionally trained practitioners at a disadvantage. In these new therapy modalities the practitioner must quickly render a diagnosis by discerning the core problem interfering with the client's current psychological functioning, especially in the interpersonal realm. And just as quickly, he or she is expected to provide direct advice, "here-and-now" interpretations, along with fashioning structured exercises for the client. These clinical practices may be abhorrent to traditionally trained practitioners but familiar to and facile for more recently trained clinicians. This may be one of the important ways that practice today is disagreeable to many senior practitioners.

There are still other ways that seasoned practitioners today may be at a disadvantage in comparison to their younger colleagues. Practitioners entering the field in recent years usually have more business savvy than did their predecessors. They also may be more socially and politically oriented. These factors are important assets in providing mental health services today. As one respondent from the Southwest pointed out:

Mental health care delivery is no longer a cottage industry in which services are provided by isolated individual practitioners. Rather than setting up individual shops, psychologists are connecting to psychiatrists and other mental providers to ensure a steady flow of customers and to get a bite out of the big dollars that are available from providing inpatient services.

There appear to be significant gender differences, with men more concerned about the financial issues and the working conditions than women (see Table 1).

Every practitioner is inundated with brochures and announcements on courses to meet the marketing demands of today's mental health services. Attending these courses takes time and energy. Many seasoned practitioners strongly object to this distraction, feeling that it gets in the way of their commitment to being a healer. Said one psychologist:

The financial, business and promoting aspects of this business are loathsome to me. I am not interested in being a businessman. I believe that all my dissatisfactions in my practice can be traced to this disdain. The clinical issues have not been major issues.

Finally, an issue that was not raised by the respondents but will clearly have considerable impact on the practice of seasoned practitioners in the near future is the shift in the funding of mental health services. As psychotherapy in the past has been integrally tied to private health insurance carriers, in the future of psychotherapy it may well be closely related to the precise type of national health insurance eventually enacted by Congress.

Question two asked:

Is psychotherapy an impossible career insofar as there are inherent limitations to therapeutic dialogue? If so, what are these limitations?

None of the respondents claimed to believe that the practice of psychotherapy is impossible. The majority emphasized that the underlying structure of therapeutic dialogue is an arena in which compassionate healing can take place. Typical is the point of view expressed by a psychiatrist from the Southwest:

> *Practicing psychotherapy is difficult but not impossible. An ongoing self-analysis and flexible approaches within ethical boundaries is the key way to ensure that therapy will be successful.*

Another psychiatrist indicated that the impediments to therapy are those inherent in any close relationship:

> *Psychotherapy is limited by therapists' clumsiness, by their inability to see beyond the limits of their own conceptual framework, and by the fact that humans are greatly flawed. It should be obvious that establishing and maintaining an intimate relationship is one of life's most difficult tasks, but the tendency of psychotherapists is to blame interpersonal disruptions on psychopathology rather than recognizing the difficulty of the task and helping individuals to view the difficulties in a positive way.*

Still other respondents maintained that the limits to therapeutic dialogue resided more in whether the patient wished to devote the time and had the money for long-term work than in the relationship itself.

On the other hand, some practitioners regarded the limitations in either the patient's psychological availability (for example, one respondent claimed that "some people can't be helped, because of early damage") or the therapist's lack of personal preparation. Said a psychoanalytically oriented psychologist:

> *The limitations are representative of the fears and grandiosity of the therapist and suggest that the practitioner had a poor personal analysis.*

Due to practical considerations such as those mentioned above, a number of respondents who expressed disappointment with their practice felt that the actual process of psychotherapy is more often a restoration of a homeostatic state between conflictual internal forces rather than a resolution of underlying psychological conflict. The homeostatic balance is quite tenuous and requires periodic psychological attention to keep conflict from violently erupting. In this regard, one of the respondents, who was strongly optimistic about his therapeutic skills when he began his career but far more cautions about them now, stated:

> *The curative powers of psychotherapy have been greatly overrated, and experienced practitioners have less of a belief that they can cure than that they help by restoring a psychic balance.*

Still other practitioners pointed out that it is the presence *of moral courage*—rather than the degree of severity and the precise nature of the patient's psychopathology, or the therapist's expertise—in conjunction with the receptiveness of the community to the patient, that is most significant in healing. In other words, it is the patient's fortitude in coming to terms with his or her condition, and to a lesser degree the therapist's courage, that enables healing to happen. Said one therapist:

> *The limits imposed by practical considerations can be disposed of if the therapist has the courage to be himself.*

From the exquisite attunement that is derived from the courage to struggle caringly together, "there are brief moments of true intimacy and understanding that make the difficult work worthwhile," said a Canadian psychologist.

I do believe that there are actually inherent limitations to therapeutic dialogue. I will discuss my view on these limitations in Chapter 7.

Question three inquired:

What do you believe to be the perils to the practitioner and the iatrogenic effects of psychotherapy to the patient?

Most of the respondents were in agreement that the most serious peril to being a clinical practitioner is the isolation of sole practice. Typical of the majority of responses to this question, one practitioner pointed out that the major consequence of the isolation of practice is that the practitioner "gets no feedback about his work."

The seasoned practitioner, even more than the beginner, lives in a solitary professional world. More than most professionals, senior psychotherapists struggle with issues and concerns alone. And also

more than in most other professions, their work is highly subjective — there are few objective standards and guidelines to be found in
the professional literature as to what constitutes successful mature
practice other than making an adequate livelihood. Even if there were
some guidelines, there are ample data to suggest that practitioners
often don't accurately report how they practice (Fiedler, 1950, 1951).
So even practitioners with some definite ideas about what constitutes
successful practice would have difficulty comparing what they do in
their consulting rooms with what their colleagues actually do.

Respondents reported that closely related to the seasoned practitioner's isolation are transference reactions by patients that are as
attractive to the therapist as they are to the patient. Confirming
Wheelis's (1956) impressionistic report of three and a half decades
ago, several practitioners pointed to the therapist's "addiction to one
directional intimacy" as one of the most serious perils to the practitioner and a leading cause of iatrogenic effects of psychotherapy.

Compromises with appropriate and ethical practice occur at those
junctures in experienced practitioners' work where their capacity for
understanding and properly evaluating the consequences of their actions has been temporarily impeded by maturational issues and personal crisis. Chessick (1990) indicates that therapists whose personal
analysis focused on traditional oedipal issues and did not sufficiently
examine pregenital and narcissistic problems are more vulnerable to
being adversely thrown by upsetting external events and the aging
process than those who gave more attention to the development of
the self. Dr. O., whose interview is discussed in Chapter 7, strongly
endorses this point of view. Not aware of their needs and how they
may be using their patients in countertherapeutic ways, practitioners
are likely to act out their narcissistic difficulties with patients at
vulnerable moments when their customary means of security and
satisfaction are strongly threatened. Even Freud was not immune: in
his advancing years, Freud's need for love and adoration was height-
ened. Storr (1983) tells us that when Freud's favorite analysand, Marie Bonaparte, revealed to him that she loved him, he made sure that
she would have two daily analytic sessions with him.

Isolation also carries with it the rampage threat of emotional
"burn-out." "There are practitioners," it was pointed out by many of
the respondents, "who are so busy looking after patients that the
perpetuation of self-sacrifice has become a way of life and they are
not able to take proper care of themselves."

According to one psychiatric practitioner, these experienced therapists may not take responsibility for their own disillusionment. Instead, "they blame their patients for these failures rather than trying to meet their patients where they are and using techniques that seem appropriate to patients as individuals."

Physical fatigue also plays a deleterious role in the mid-life of these practitioners. A psychiatrist in the full-time practice of psychoanalysis reports:

> *I didn't figure on getting tired in mid-afternoon or know what aging was about. That's a tough one to anticipate in any profession. I underrated the sitting.*

This physical discomfort is underscored by a female psychologist who says that the need to sit back and listen to a great deal of pain and unhappiness all day and into the evening results in actually feeling "severe physical pain" in her back when she tries to relax at home in the evening. It seems as if the requirement for a high degree of empathy and understanding can force a bodily passivity which contains denied and held-in strong feelings of the therapist.

For many of the respondents these held-in feelings may consist of adverse reactions to the business of practicing psychotherapy. When asked about the perils of practice, one experienced practitioner indicated that the wear-and-tear on the therapist's health was a direct result of "the temptation to long hours because of a need for money."

The continual onslaught of physically and psychically painful work has for many therapists resulted in disillusionment about their involvement as psychotherapists. One seasoned practitioner indicated that in his experience therapists who suffer from disillusionment about the nature and meaningfulness of their work respond in an either/or way. Rather than "taking their work appropriately seriously, they either regard what they do as trivial or, on the other hand, are overly serious and heavy about their practices." In regard to therapists who experience being a practitioner negatively, a midwest psychologist indicated:

> . . . *the therapist can develop a coldness and pedantic defenses against his feelings or, occasionally, can get overinvolved with a patient.*

To the extent that practitioners get disillusioned Table 1 suggests that male practitioners are more likely than female practitioners to perceive this as an ethical or moral issue.

One of the most difficult and dangerous overinvolvements, which raises serious ethical and moral issues, comes from working with an "as if" patient/colleague. In an extended report, one of the respondents discussed the perilous therapeutic work with such a patient.

The caring and concerned senior practitioner, if he is willing to work with difficult patients, will be approached for assistance by colleagues who are in severe personal and professional conflict. It is complimentary to be asked to serve in this capacity; it also can be rather dangerous. Because of the patient's unrecognized shame about his incompetence, he will be approaching the practitioner not so much for therapeutic assistance as for confirmation that even highly skilled colleagues have flaws and limitations. The respondent who reported his work with an "as if" colleague indicated that his patient, Dr. M., evinced an unwitting magical belief that, if the "as if" colleague/patient could find from firsthand experience serious limitations in his highly respected therapist, then he would be absolved of personal responsibility for his own actions and the need to come to terms with his character problems. The unfortunate consequences of working with dangerous colleagues is discussed in Chapter 8.

In an important political sense, psychotherapists are given *privilege*. They are rewarded with status and high fees in return for the personal temperament and skills to withstand behaviors that are intolerable to ordinary people. The question that needs to be answered is the extent to which practitioners differ in their ability and willingness to deal with the dilemmas of their clinical practice. One of the assumptions upon which depends the representativeness of the findings of this study is that seasoned practitioners from different backgrounds from those in my study respond similarly to the issues, concerns, and dilemmas of psychotherapeutic practice as do my respondents.

An overall question important to ask in terms of the perils of practice for experienced therapists, therefore, is how representative my respondents are of practitioners at large. To address this concern, I compared what experienced practitioners reported to me to the findings of a heterogenous sample of psychotherapists who discussed the stresses and satisfactions of their psychotherapeutic work in a previous study. Farber and Heifetz (1981, 1982) administered three Likert-type rating inventories to sixty practitioners — psychologists, psychiatrists and social workers — drawn from a Northeastern metropolitan community of approximately 350,000 people.

A factor analysis of the data from this investigation revealed that the most stressful factors of those studied included feeling "personally depleted by therapeutic work, coping with pressures inherent in the therapeutic relationship, and dealing with difficult working conditions." The most satisfying aspects of therapeutic work were "promoting personal growth and change, achieving intimate involvement in the lives of patients, and feeling professionally respected." Farber and Heifetz (1982) concluded that the respondents expected clinical work to be difficult and stressful and were willing to put up with the adverse effects of their work to the extent that their efforts appeared to "pay off." When they didn't receive success and recognition they believed to be proportional to their efforts, however, these practitioners reported feeling debilitated and "burnt out."

My respondents seem highly consistent with those practitioners investigated by Farber and Heifetz. This finding serves to give some consensual validation to the study reported here.

Question four asked:

Have you ever struggled with whether to return to the "couch"? If so, what enabled you to resolve this issue?

This item was an indirect attempt to tap the respondents' feelings about their personal analysis or therapy at various points in their careers. There were two basic responses to this issue. One grouping consisted of psychoanalytically oriented practitioners, predominantly psychiatrists, who appeared from their responses on other questionnaire items to have minimally changed their views about neurosis and clinical practice through the years. These respondents reported that they had excellent personal therapies and still respected their analysts and the work they did with them even after many years. Typical of this attitude is that of a psychiatrist with over forty years experience as a practitioner:

I had 4+ years of psychoanalysis by an eminent New York analyst to whom I have a remaining positive transference and who has confirmed my admiration by his scientific contributions throughout the years after I completed analysis.

Practitioners of this persuasion report returning for additional therapy as no struggle. Said one such respondent:

It wasn't a struggle, I returned at various crisis or change points in my life, for example, divorce and remarriage.

Said another analyst respondent:

Every therapist should return and return.

Other respondents with highly favorable reactions to their own personal therapy indicated that a number of practical factors have prevented their returning for more than a brief "revisiting." The primary factors mentioned were the large expenditures of time and money required for a second analysis. And while a second analysis seems appealing at times, one psychologist said, "So are many other activities."

For the highly experienced practitioner still another factor is important. Said a respondent:

I have only returned in special situations. These were situations that involved my conflictual relationship with my wife and later with a woman with whom I was living. In these instances, I sought out conjoint therapy. The reason is that not only is it difficult to ask help for myself alone, but there is also some grandiosity on my part in not being able to find a therapist who is at least my peer.

Correspondingly, a New York psychologist with thirty-five years of clinical experience revealed:

There were only two therapists I would have gone to and one is dead; the other has moved to Boston and isn't available anymore for me. But then, I question if I need more personal therapy experience. I believe that I understand most of what I go through. It's really hard to fool myself about myself for very long, even when I symptomatize.

What are the life experiences that best enable practitioners to understand themselves meaningfully and satisfyingly? Most people would take for granted that this would inevitably follow from the practitioner's personal analysis or therapy. I should point out, however, that several of the prominent psychotherapists who revealed their personal thoughts to Burton (1972) called this assumption into serious question. They were disappointed, some even bitter, about their experiences in personal analysis. They indicated that during their careers they had found life experiences far more rewarding than their own analyses. One of the most important findings of my study is that this discontentment about personal therapy is supported by a considerable number of the experienced practitioners who were involved in my investigation. They claimed to have profited more from encounters with their patients, supervision, peer consultation, and nonclinical experiences than from their personal analysis or therapy. Typical of this attitude, a psychologist on the East Coast said:

> *Contacts with colleagues and family have kept me off the couch.*

Similarly, a psychiatrist from the Southwest admitted:

> *When I have wished for someone to speak with intimately I have someone available. One of my grown sons is someone I frequently have turned to.*

For quite a few of the very experienced practitioners, spiritual reawakening has meant more to them throughout their years as therapists than their earlier experiences in personal therapy. Said one respondent:

> *I don't have too much faith in most therapists helping me. Instead, I have opened myself up to a wide range of Eastern philosophies and Western spiritual messages.*

Other respondents speak of having learned to take better care of themselves, not from personal therapy but from self-analysis and from help and consultation by friends and colleagues. Representative of this method for self-monitoring, a Midwest psychiatrist indicated:

> *I'm in self-analysis and peer supervision (for two hours at a minimum a week).*

Others speak of experiences from their private lives as having provided an impetus for taking better care of themselves. One of the dominant themes in the responses of practitioners who, instead of returning to the couch, have turned to books, spiritual inspiration, friendship, and family involvement is the insight that when they were less mature they suffered from a need to be unstintingly available to their patients at a severe cost to their own and their family's well-being. Today, they are no longer as unrealistically flexible to patient demands as they were earlier in their careers. Patient needs, they report, are now balanced with their own needs and those of their families.

Question five asked:

What has been your experience with self-analysis?

This question examines the nature of the obstacles in the way of self-knowledge.

The Socratic doctrine "Know thyself!" is the ethos of our profession. Our clinical training is built upon the belief that, to the extent that self-understanding is ignored, our clinical competence will be compromised and our personal lives unfulfilled. Practitioners' self-examination is crucial to their patients' progress, not only because it enables therapists to recognize how their own issues may be interfering with their reception and understanding of what their patients are reporting, but also because the patient's presentation alone is insufficient for a complete understanding of what the patient is intending to communicate. Rumination from the practitioner's psyche augments the patient's presentation (Reik, 1964).

The mandate of understanding the sufferer's problems from the practitioner's insight into his or her own is a basic tenant of the healing tradition. From earliest time practitioners have created healing systems for those they treat in terms of the meanings they have made of their own suffering and life crises. These are meanings they have come across in their own self-examination. Practitioners who feel that they know themselves "well enough" from their personal therapy will find their work rather dull and mechanical. Unless practitioners are still curious in examining their lives after completing personal treatment, they will feel restless and bored with their daily clinical tasks. With these considerations in mind, Freud (1937) regarded self-examination to be indispensable to the most profound understanding of any problem and recommended that the psychotherapist continue a regular process of self-analysis after the practitioner's personal analysis was completed. According to Jones (1961), because Freud considered his own search for self-knowledge to be a process that could never be wisely dispensed with, Freud religiously attended his own self-analysis the last hour of each day.

According to Fleming (1971), from Freud's original training pro-

posal for future practitioners, one of the primary objectives of psychotherapeutic training to this day is to foster a lifelong commitment
to self-analysis through the processes of "introspection, empathy, and
interpretation." Yet, despite its core property in psychotherapeutic
education, precise procedures for how to go about conducting one's
own analysis or self-examination are neglected in both the psychoanalytic and psychotherapy literatures. In his review on the literature of
self-analysis Chessick (1990) indicates that no analyst he has ever
read has actually described what goes on in the process of self-analysis in terms of the interminable and multimotivational sources of the
uncovered material. More recently, Sonnenberg (1991), an analyst,
has attempted to address these missing descriptions by focusing on
the details of his own self-analysis over a period of several months
following an illness in his aged mother.

Personal vignettes by a few practitioners will not, of course, provide us with the rate of overall utilization of self-examination among
psychotherapists, nor will they furnish us with information about
how useful psychotherapists-in-general have found their efforts at
self-examination. The usefulness and the limitations of self-analysis
can be best answered by a representative sample of those who have
practiced it the most faithfully for the longest period of time. The
respondents in my study would appear to fulfill this criterion.

Tables 3 and 4 provide information in terms of gender and professional affiliation about the usefulness of self-analysis for experienced
psychotherapists.

Does the commitment to self-analysis have the same value for my
respondents as it was reported to have had for experienced practitioners in the past? As we can see from Tables 3 and 4, more of the
respondents had positive experience with self-analysis than negative.
Typically, one respondent said:

*Self-analysis, whatever you want to call it, is critical to excellence in
clinical performance.*

However, rather than being an ongoing routine of their clinical
preparation, self-examination appears to be used at especially trying
times in their lives. Said a New York psychologist:

*I do this but not formally—usually when I feel stressed about some-
thing and not as a routine exercise.*

TABLE 3: Experience with Self-Analysis

Attitude	Males (37)		Females (15)		Total	
	n	%	n	%	n	%
Very positive	1	2.7	1	6.7	2	3.8
Positive	15	40.5	5	33.3	20	38.5
Ambivalent	7	18.9	4	26.7	11	21.2
Negative	9	24.3	3	20	12	23.1
Not able to determine from respondent's statement	5	13.5	2	13.3	7	13.5

Few reported self-examination to have been of great value for understanding significant issues, as Freud (1900) claimed for his self-analytic efforts. Said one Chicago respondent:

It has some value, but I often keep bumping into the same bumps.

A psychologist from the Northwest indicated:

Usually works well so long as it is a relatively minor issue.

One eminent psychiatrist from the Midwest referred to the process of self-analysis as "ridiculous!" In short, many of the respondents seem to agree with Chessick's (1990) assessment that "the issue of self-analysis after one's training psychoanalysis is turning out to be

TABLE 4: Experience with Self-Analysis

Attitude	Psychiatrists (15)		Psychologists (33)		Social Workers (4)	
	n	%	n	%	n	%
Very positive	1	6.7	1	3.0	0	0
Positive	4	26.7	15	45.5	1	25
Ambivalent	3	20	8	24.2	0	0
Negative	4	26.7	6	18.2	2	50
Not able to determine	3	20	4	12.1	0	0

much more complicated than originally thought." In fact, in light of my finding, Chessick's comment may be an understatement.

A second important finding of the study is that, in addition to those who have ambivalent experiences with self-examination, there is a considerable number of respondents who actually have negative attitudes about self-analysis. They report that they cannot proceed in areas of psychological investigation where resistances have not previously been removed by personal therapy. These practitioners report having encountered formidable and often insurmountable obstacle in trying to continue self-examination after individual therapy. Their attempts to understand their psychic processes, they report, result in sterile intellectual forays. Admits a psychologist from the Midwest:

I never developed any great skill with it, despite personal analysis.

Correspondingly, a psychologist from the West Coast wrote:

Self-examination is OK within the usual limits. However, there always is the danger of overintellectualization and hyper self-centeredness.

In many instances successfully coming to terms with one's suffering requires the recognition that one feels alone in struggling with one's burdens because one has become alienated from the caring and concern of others. The need to recognize the subtly detrimental role that an overattachment to self-examination may be playing in a practitioner's life is stated by one psychologist as follows:

Self-examination may be very helpful. For me it has even been lifesaving. But it cannot stand on its own for too long. It requires a sharing of its findings with others to foster a fuller understanding of its import. Indeed, for a practitioner to act obsessively on the belief that self-analysis is the royal road, while others are temporary walkways, contradicts the essential interpersonal dimension of all psychotherapies.

Because in self-examination it is too easy to fool oneself, most of the practitioners in this study reported that they worked with friends and supervisors and regularly attended peer consultation and even therapy groups for themselves in which their "blind spots" could be more propitiously examined than in self-analysis. Freud, as is well-known, reviewed the speculative findings of his self-analysis with a trusted friend, the strange physician Wilhelm Fliess. We should applaud his pioneering efforts as courageous and forthright (though perhaps misdirected in the case of Fliess). Practitioners today, as I will discuss in Chapter 9, are in a more fortunate position with regard to broaching their own painful issues.

Question six asked:

Have your views on neurosis and human nature changed during your career? If so, how?

In keeping with the previously mentioned dichotomy of therapist responses, there were two clusters of perspectives on this question. Most of the respondents reported that over the years they have greatly changed their world views. They are less grandiose about their skills. They regard themselves less *the crucial* agent of change and more as a useful facilitative agent. Changes in one's view of neurosis and human nature are strongly affected by one's understanding of human suffering. The need to change their views about human behavior came from their gradual recognition that their clinical training had been directed by misguided clinical theories. The considerable dissatisfaction with clinical theory is the third major finding of the study. As Table 1 suggests, male practitioners seem significantly more concerned with the limitations of their theoretical preparation than do female therapists.

These practitioners, both males and females, currently have a greater respect for and a firmer faith in their patients' healing capacities than in the past. A New York psychiatrist indicates:

Have I changed my views? And how! I understand people and neurosis in a way that was simply opaque twenty years ago. Not that it's clear, but I see enough to help in a more direct, efficient way. Twenty years ago, the patient had to do all the work.

Because they themselves have lived more fully, they are now less captive of the authority of abstract theory—which is actually the distillation of other practitioners' experiences, presented as universal occurrence.

Another New York practitioner reports that she now

. . . sees people as continually evolving and seeking their own awareness. I view all behavior as essentially positive and purposive. I do not

discriminate between neurotic and normal behavior as we were taught
in the past. I treat patients on the same basis as I want to be treated.

Other respondents traced their present change in attitude from
moving "from a disease model to one of increased awareness of social
oppression, prejudice and family dysfunction." Correspondingly, still
other practitioners emphasized the existential and narcissistic issues
of intimate bonding rather than the moral masochistic intrapsychic
preoccupation of patients, as was emphasized in their early clinical
training. One respondent reported that she now recognizes a wider
range of patient behavior that is adaptive rather than pathological
than when she was younger. To this we can add the statement of a
prominent Swiss psychiatrist and analyst who indicated that:

Whereas in former times I saw more infantile conflicts as the origins of
neurosis, I recognize now more deficiency experiences due to the lack
of love and sufficient attention or due to an overprotective attitude as
the causes of neurosis.

For still other practitioners who have radically modified their views
of human suffering, these beliefs have been transformed from

. . . traditional psychodynamics to a more spiritual view—inner
peace, forgiveness, compassion—which come from the willingness of
the therapist to give up anger and resentment in the foolish belief that
it will protect self-integrity.

Accompanying their own increased tolerance for the frailties of
human nature has been the fostering of more relaxed, flexible, and
responsive ways of working with patients. One practitioner indicated
that his view of human nature had "softened and mellowed." A
Washington, D.C. psychologist indicated that she has

. . . come to rely much more on the strengths and the responses of
even quite sick people.

In response to greater tolerance of individuals' idiosyncratic ways
of relating to the demands of human existence, there appears to be
some resignation to the tenacity of some human problems, but reluctance to hammer away at them in the righteous way the practitioner
had done in the past. Philosophically, this was expressed by a Southwest psychiatrist, who indicated that he has come to realize that

. . . humans are not so much good or evil as they are a potpourri of banal motivations: to eat and sleep comfortably; to achieve recognition from peers; to have comfortable relationships and satisfying work. To keep ourselves going, we glorify the banal, and it works.

In rather sharp contrast, the second type of response to this question of whether their view of human nature and neurosis had changed consisted of statements indicating that these experienced therapists had "more respect for defenses and the power and entrenchment of neurosis" and they were "less idealistic about growth possibilities" than they had been as beginners. These practitioners, in reflecting on the human condition, sadly concluded that

. . . some people will never change. Therapy just is not for everyone. I once thought that it was.

A couple of the most senior practitioners who answered the questionnaire indicated that their views about human nature and neurosis had not changed substantially over the years; the reason for this will be discussed in Chapter 10.

Question seven asked:

What have been the most important lessons you have learned from your patients?

In important aspects the responses to this question followed from the answers that the respondents gave to the previous question about their changing views of human nature. These professionals for the most part admitted that they were as interested in personal growth as they were in patient growth; consequently, the lessons of clinical practice represent personal insights. Almost all reported positive personal gains from their work with patients. "Each patient offers a whole new world to learn from," said one respondent. Others pointed to "the recognition of how identical we are to our patients" in what we experience in trying to come to terms with our human condition. These insights have led some practitioners to develop a greater capacity for:

humility, patience, a need for flexibility and clarity about one's own values, ethics, and spirituality.

It underscored in still other practitioners:

> *the value of a sense of humor, the importance of presence in human encounter (based on the willingness to listen deeply and be humble) and a deeply grounded affirmation of life that is conducive to their trusting their patients' determination to survive meaningfully.*

This may be summarized in the statement of one practitioner who has come to realize that his patients are far wiser than he had assumed. He also has come to recognize that there is no single, objectively true reality. Therefore,

> *. . . confronting patients with what the practitioner believes to be their invalid reality is not too helpful. Realities are separate and multiple. The important therapeutic question is which of these "realities" is most functional to the patient in terms of what the patient is willing and able to commit him/herself to responsibly.*

Question eight inquired:

What effect has being a psychotherapist had on your relationship with family, friends and a sense of community?

A safe haven at home, close relationships, interesting activities and involvements outside of practice seem vital for the practitioner. The times of greatest stress for therapists generally are those in which they must face the daily onslaught of their patients' emotional issues without experiencing that their own emotional needs are being adequately met.

Tables 5 and 6 indicate the effect of being a practitioner on significant people in the respondents' personal lives. They show a bimodal configuration to what the effect of being a psychotherapist had on private life. Overall, for one grouping the result has been decidedly positive. Said one respondent:

> *It has been necessary for me to build strong friendships, family ties and linkages with community projects in order to be effective and not burn out.*

Reported another practitioner:

TABLE 5: Effects of Being a Practitioner on Significant Others

Effect	Males (31)		Females (15)		Total	
	n	%	n	%	n	%
Positive	15	40.5	3	20	18	34.6
Ambivalent	9	24.3	1	6.7	10	19.2
Negative	12	32.4	7	46.7	19	36.5
Not able to determine	3	8.1	2	13.3	5	9.6

It has deepened my sense of what it means to be connected to the human race and to particular people. It has given me a sense of responsibility to share with the community.

Still another practitioner indicated:

Being a therapist certainly has helped me with my family. I've changed some of my earlier concepts about relationships. With family and friends I have been more open about my feelings and willing to trust them than when I was younger.

In contrast, many of the respondents report that being a therapist has certain built-in limitations to friendship and community involvement. This is the fourth important finding. Combining the negative and ambivalent categories we find that more practitioners saw an adverse effect of being a therapist on their relationships with signifi-

TABLE 6: Effects of Being a Practitioner on Significant Others

Effect	Psychi-atrists (15)		Psychol-ogists (33)		Social Workers (4)	
	n	%	n	%	n	%
Positive	5	33.3	13	39.4	1	25
Ambivalent	5	33.3	5	15.2	0	0
Negative	4	26.7	13	39.4	2	50
Not able to determine	1	6.7	2	6.1	1	25

cant others than those who perceived a positive influence. One practitioner admitted that

. . . it is fortunate that I have close friends who are therapists. I don't speak with nontherapist friends about my work, except in generalities. As a result, I haven't developed any strong sense of community.

The sense of alienation from family and friends caused by the long hours and severe demands of practice, especially when one works with a number of seriously disturbed patients at the same time, was underscored by several respondents. Said one:

Being a practitioner has kept me a little apart in social situations.

Said a New York psychiatrist, reflecting on earlier times in his career:

Unfortunately, the demands of my career and my studies at the New York Psychoanalytic Institute deprived my son and daughter of time I would have liked to have spent with them from the time they were infants up to age eight.

The lack of involvement, another New York analyst indicated, may be due to how dull the world outside the consulting room seems in contrast to what happens inside. He goes on to say:

The work of psychoanalysis is a fascinating job. But there is a certain danger that after work an interest in other relationships diminishes and that as a result of this there is a certain isolation and even a neglect of family.

Still other practitioners admitted, perhaps shamefully, that being a therapist did not increase their sensitivity to family. In terms of their children, a few suggested that being a practitioner had a paradoxical influence on their relationship with them. They confessed to being unreasonably unsympathetic and intolerant with their own children's failures. Said one child psychologist:

I seem to do better with other people's children. Mine don't seem to speak to me as easily as other children do.

Because of the tendency to pathologize and to see things in relationships that other people don't, some of the respondents wrote that they have had to be especially careful in not revealing to friends and family what they see going on in social situations.

Practitioners who can't share professional concerns with family and friends may become insulated from them. In these instances patients who share similar issues and concerns may become increasingly more attractive and important to the isolated practitioner, as the story of Nora in Chapter 2 illustrated. There may be many Noras in our profession. This is suggested from the research of Henry and his associates (1971), who found that, for most of the therapists studied, relationships with patients were more emotionally intense and satisfying than affliations with spouses and children. We all know of senior practitioners for whom patients have become home, family, mission, and destiny. It was said of Harry Stack Sullivan, as I was told while I was in analytic training in the Washington School of Psychiatry which was housed in Sullivan's former townhouse in downtown Washington, D.C., that his patients were his closest companions. Apparently, at various times several of them even boarded with him in his large townhouse.

In terms of gender there appear to be clear differences on question 8. In general, being a practitioner has a decisively more negative effect on female practitioners than males in regard to their relationships with significant others.

Question nine inquired:

Have there been satisfactions in your practice that you had not antici-pated as a beginner? If so, what are they?

If one is to continue practicing psychotherapy there have to be satisfactions to neutralize the distress and discontentment encountered in working with human suffering. In general, in addition to being able to make a good livelihood, the satisfactions of therapeutic practice derive from what the practitioner's life history and psychic disposition have impelled him or her toward—the opportunity and competence to explore with others the mysteries of human existence by means of a highly personal experience.

Tables 7 and 8 list by category respondents' reports of the unanticipated satisfactions of being a psychotherapist, differentiating among them in terms of gender and professional affiliation.

For the most part, the respondents reported that their satisfactions were those that they had anticipated but had not quite appreciated as

TABLE 7: Unanticipated Satisfactions

Satisfaction	Males (37)		Females (15)		Total	
	n	%	n	%	n	%
Self-development	15	40.1	7	46.7	22	42.3
Social	13	35.1	4	26.7	17	32.7
Altruistic	10	27.0	3	20	13	25
Creative	5	13.5	2	13.3	7	13.5
Financial and working conditions	4	10.8	1	6.7	5	9.6
Being part of a therapeutic community	3	8.1	0	0	3	5.8

a younger person. Many mentioned that the greatest satisfactions came from enjoying intimacy and closeness with patients that they had not experienced with anyone before. Several indicated that being a healer brought out qualities in themselves of which they had some awareness but which had not been tested under fire earlier in their lives. For example, one practitioner stated:

> *Altruism was not an interest that I had believed that I held in high esteem when I was younger. But I have become more comfortable with just being human and becoming aware of needing the same kinds of things as other people do—including the need to be cooperative and of help to others.*

Some expressed their satisfactions quite evocatively:

TABLE 8: Unanticipated Satisfaction

Satisfaction	Psychiatrists (15)		Psychologists (33)		Social Workers (4)	
	n	%	n	%	n	%
Self-development	7	46.7	13	39.4	2	50
Social	1	6.7	15	45.5	1	25
Altruistic	4	26.7	8	24.2	1	25
Creative	2	13.3	5	15.2	0	0
Financial and working conditions	1	6.7	3	9.1	1	25
Political	2	13.3	1	3.0	0	0

The "rush" of being a player in the enhancement of another is even more pleasurable than I had imagined, with its sense of power and competence when therapy goes well.

Some practitioners expressed their satisfactions as senior therapists quite lyrically and visually; for example, one respondent said:

Watching the growth of some patients has been like a flower opening and blooming. It sometimes takes your breath away.

Other practitioners expressed their satisfactions quite modestly:

Just getting little "thank you" cards after treatment or having patients come back after many years to say "hello" and to tell me that we accomplished something important is what it is all about for me.

There appear to be gender differences in regard to the unanticipated satisfactions of practice. This impression is based on applying cultural expectations about male and female role behavior in contemporary United States to the data. Table 7 shows male and female practitioners deriving unanticipated satisfactions from altruistic, social, and emotional self-developmental activities in their practice in approximate proportions to their representation in the research sample. In our culture, however, women are more predominantly involved in these activities than are men. One might therefore expect women to be more highly represented in these categories than Table 7 indicates. When I asked how they would explain this finding, two of the female practitioners interviewed (see Chapter 7) suggested that, because women play these roles in so many nontherapy settings, the rewards are not unanticipated and need not be emphasized as professional satisfactions. To the extent that this perception is accurate, it is the fifth significant finding of this study.

There also appears to be significant differences between psychologists and psychiatrists in regard to some of the unanticipated satisfactions of practice. Psychologists placed a higher value on the social and interpersonal aspects of clinical practice than did the psychiatrists. This may be due to the fact that the psychologists in this study are more interpersonally interactive than the psychiatrists and therefore enjoyed the opportunity for more interpersonal satisfaction. It also could be attributed to a temperamentally greater need of the psychologists for interpersonal interaction than their psychiatric colleagues. There is insufficient data to assess whether there are marked differences in either the personalities or clinical methodology of the practitioners studied. However, there is another possibility for which there is some evidence. It may be that the practitioners studied as a group have similar social and interpersonal needs, but that psychologists need to satisfy this interest in clinical practice because, as Table 6 suggests, they find that being a practitioner has more of a negative effect for them than it does for psychiatrists in maintaining significant relationships with family, friends and community. If valid, this finding in regard to psychologists is in agreement with the evidence that Henry and his associates' large study (1971) provided that practitioners of each of the major mental health professions tend as a group to have warmer and closer relationships with their patients than with family and friends.

Question ten asked:

Do you have a "personal myth" that has directed the way you practice and how you live your life? If so, what is it? If it has changed during your career, how has it done so?

For the most part, respondents denied the importance of a personal myth in their lives. Apparently many of them did not understand what I meant by the term. Still others regarded a personal myth as something negative, like poor reality-testing. For example, one practitioner referred to a personal myth as "representing the danger of submitting to an ideology." Another regarded it as the conflictual baggage he carried for most of his career and now had finally rid himself of in his private life, as well as in his clinical work.

It is unfortunate for practitioners not to recognize the critical role personal myths play in human existence (Bagarozzi and Anderson, 1989). It is extremely important that we get closely in touch with what we unwittingly assume will happen as a result of our becoming therapists. Our own personal myths offer us one of the most expedient means of capturing what being a therapist means to us.

It is intrinsic to human existence to regard the events of one's life evaluatively. We are meaning-oriented beings. One's personal identity is constituted in ways expressed by the *stories one tells oneself* about what has happened in one's life. Each of us has, if not a favorite story about oneself, then at least a prototypic story that has direct implications for how we regard the world, its resources, opportunities, and impediments to the achievement of our desires. These stories derive from a wide range of sources. Since we cannot empirically acquire absolute truth about our world, each of us attempts, by using the events, legends, and myths of family and society, to create a reliable guide for living (Goldberg, 1991).

The practitioner who wishes to become enlightened must rediscover and assimilate precisely those basic "archetypical images," as Jung (1956) called them, contained in universal myths. Examining the obstacles in the seeker's path in terms of the symbolic meaning of enduring myths uncovers viable options for understanding human experience and sharing the spiritual tradition with those who have preceded the seeker. These symbols have inspired people through the millennia to face the longings and suffering of the human psyche with courage, compassion, and vision. This is to say, once the seeker starts a personal journey in search of enlightenment, he or she joins a venerable human endeavor (Goldberg, 1990b).

Those respondents who seemed to understand what I meant by personal myth either wrote of their own personal myth as a recognizable societal myth (for example, the myth of Sisyphus) or stated it in everyday terms, "You have to work hard to be successful," "I see myself as a vehicle helping passersby," or "He who saves one life saves the world."

Question eleven inquired:

What does the term "master therapist" mean to you?

Some respondents wrote that they had never heard the term used before. Most others regarded the term as a negative expression for a practitioner who is a self-promoter. Cynically, perhaps, one New York practitioner wrote:

A master therapist is a pompous ass, who does therapy tapes of his brilliant successes and lies about his failures.

(He mentioned a couple of very prominent theorists, who he regarded in this pejorative way.)

A few of the respondents defined a master therapist as a practitioner who has exceptional therapeutic and teaching skills. This attitude is exemplified in a psychiatrist's statement:

Master therapists have a thorough indoctrination in the theories and techniques of what they do, recognize the limitations of these theories and techniques, and know that each individual has the potential for having an entirely separate experience, requiring an altogether different way of looking at the world.

Finally, question twelve asked for:

Those books and articles that you found the most helpful in shaping your work as a psychotherapist.

The composite of basic literature as indicated by the respondents' selections appears to reflect a lack of general agreement on the value of contributions to the psychotherapy profession.

I will not try to cover all the literary works mentioned, only those listed by at least four respondents. In this regard, it was not surprising that Sigmund Freud's writings were most often mentioned. However, that they were "most helpful" to only eleven of the practitioners, who were almost all psychodynamically oriented, was not something I would have anticipated. In second place was Harry Stack Sullivan, with seven listings, then D. W. Winnicott with six listings. Frieda Fromm-Reichmann, Harold Searles and Theodor Reik were impressive for five of the respondents. Heinz Kohut, Allen Wheelis, and Jay Haley all received four mentions. Among other works mentioned, including the Old Testament, the Talmud, the works of Shakespeare and other literary classics, and the writings of spiritual masters of various persuasions, none received more than three votes.

There were some notable omissions. I would have expected the works of Carl G. Jung, Erik Erikson, Anna Freud, and Otto Kernberg to be more prominently mentioned. However, again I need to remind the reader that my selection of therapists questioned was not random and may not represent the views of most senior practitioners. It is quite possible that experienced practitioners at large would respond differently from those queried in my study. It also should be noted that the writings were selected in retrospect. In my case, at different times in my career I would have chosen different authors as important.

Before ending this chapter, let me offer a few words of recommendation for further investigation of mature practice. While trends are apparent in the information reported in this pilot study, the sample was too small to allow for a statistical analysis. A larger sample would enable us to more clearly perceive important trends in the information reported. It would be useful if this sample were comprised of male and female practitioners of different professional affiliations, ethnic and racial groups, and cultural and religious membership comparable to their representation in professional practice. Moreover, in that seasoned practitioners may range in age from their mid-thirties to beyond their seventies, representatives of different ages should be included.

The question of the effect of the practitioner's age on the issues of significant concern deserves a brief discussion. In this book I emphasize the developmental issues of mid-life. Clearly, some of the practitioners given questionnaires and most of the prominent practitioners interviewed are beyond middle age. Developmental theory tells us that the maturational issues differ in senior maturity from those of mid-life. A comparison of the concerns of practitioners from these different age groups would seem to be in order. Unfortunately, my questionnaire does not ask for the respondent's age. However, with a few exceptions this information can be inferred by using the number of years of clinical practice as a rough gauge.

I assumed that most psychotherapists start their clinical practice between the ages of twenty-five and thirty. Using Levinson et al.'s (1978) criterion of mid-life beginning between the ages of thirty-five and forty, I placed the respondents with less than fifteen years of clinical practice in the pre-midlife category. Only two respondents fell in this group. I found that twenty-six practitioners had between fifteen and thirty years of clinical experience and placed them in the mid-life category. Finally, twenty-four respondents were found to have had over thirty years of clinical experience.

Examining the issues of significant concern to the respondents by age group, I found few differences between the mid-life group and the more senior practitioners. For example, one might expect the more senior practitioners to be concerned with retirement. But it was one of the mid-life practitioners who mentioned this issue as significant. The one category that may indicate a significant difference among the three groups is that of countertransference, with which the mid-life group seemed more concerned than either of the other two.

Finally, it should be evident after reviewing the data in this chapter that the questions asked in further studies of therapist maturity should be stated in a way that enables the investigator to quantify the information and apply statistical analysis. In this study only four of the questions produced quantifiable data.

Chapter 7 discusses interviews with twelve analysts in which the findings discussed in this chapter are further developed.

In the next chapter I discuss current theories of adult development in order to create a context from to examine issues of wisdom and maturity in Chapters 7, 8, and 10.

six

ADULT DEVELOPMENT: THE TASKS OF MID-LIFE AND THE YEARS BEYOND

Who has driven the light out of my world?
What has happened to the warm, protected and rejoicing
   days promised to me in my youth?
Where have gone the summers of pride if I chose the
   virtuous life?
They have vanished like lost sands into a starless night.
I seek to return to innocence so that I might again taste
   the fruits that seemed so much the promise of my
   youthful dreams.
I cannot return to innocence.
I know cynically too much.
I am too imbued with the compromises I must undergo
   in every encounter in life to taste afresh their fruits.
Who has driven the day out of my world?

                —Carl Goldberg, 1980

In writing this book I was reminded of important mentors and friends from my youth. Countless times I told myself, "One of these days I will look up this person and write or call." What I kept denying in my procrastination was that these friends older than I were not immortal. What is not said or done today may be forever lost.

Roger Gould (1978) has written of the painful paradox of mid-life. By this season most of us are in a commanding position socially and have achieved success in our professional pursuits. We are experienced by others, if not by ourselves, as powerful in the world. Looking around, we are impressed with the realization that the world belongs to us and those of our generation. Yet all is not right with us. The disturbing vulnerabilities and depressed vitality of our bodies, together with the increasing acceleration of the loss of those people who were close to us—indeed, even those of our generation—

startlingly awaken us to the realization that something is amiss with our lives — something urgent is quickly slipping away. We sadly discover that the vitality of early adulthood has been carried off with the departure of our third decade. No one in mid-life can confidently believe that his social and professional successes will render him out of the reaches of disabling disease or emotional despair. Neurosis, addiction, and death in those we know intimately are a daily part of our world. We become aware of the tragic sense of unfulfilled hopes and aspirations of those who have fallen victim to these misfortunes. In turn, we are confronted with a sense of unfinished business in our own lives. Gould (1978) reminds us:

> The desire for stability and continuity that characterized our thirties is being replaced by a relentless inner demand for action. The sense of timelessness in our early thirties is giving way to an awareness of the pressure of time in our forties. *Whatever we must do must be done now.* (p. 217)

What specifically must we do at this time in our lives? Given the relative lack of research on mid-life, compared with the extensive research investigating childhood, adolescence, and early adulthood, the answer depends on whose personality theory you wish to follow. The theory of personality evolving from classical psychoanalysis discouraged developmental exploration of adulthood. It employed clinical evidence to demonstrate that adulthood, with rare exception, is the recreation of childhood issues. Maturity in adulthood, analytic theory posited, was made possible by the successful resolution of the psychosexual conflicts of the preoedipal and oedipal periods of childhood. While classical psychoanalytic theory dominated psychology in the first half of this century, Jungian theory has gained prominence in the second half. This is particularly true of the influence of Jungian concepts on the theoretical formulations of those psychologists today who are interested in adult development.

According to Carl Jung (1956), the ultimate goal of personality is to achieve a state of selfhood and self-realization. The self, according to Jung, is an archetype that acts as the nucleus of personality development. Jung also believed that the archetype for selfhood usually lies dominant until about middle age, which he described as beginning between the ages of thirty-five and forty. Until this time, most people have focused their existential perspective and vital energies outward. That is to say, they usually have been too preoccupied with trying to come to terms with the realities of the external world to concern themselves with the creative and spiritual needs of their inner being. At mid-life the person has, more or less, come to terms with the social and material demands on his being. For most people this means having separated from their family of origin and provided for oneself a means of livelihood and the creation of a new family. At mid-life, Jung tells us, the person is ready to *individuate*, by becoming far more aware than ever before of who he or she is as a person and of the creative and spiritual needs that he or she has without awareness yearned to fulfill. In individuation, the person's major task is to question and recast core beliefs and values. In doing this one asks oneself: Where have I been? Where am I now? Where can I reach in the time I have remaining? (Jung, 1989).

A second highly influential theorist of adult development is Erik Erikson. Following Jung's path but with a Freudian map to describe the terrain, Erikson (1950) formulated a psychological theory to describe personality development from the cradle to senior maturity. Erikson, like Jung, believes that personality development is a lifetime assignment, one that does not cease with an oedipal resolution in childhood. His work is based on the principle that anything that grows has a ground plan. The parts arising from this epigenesis have their own particular time of ascendency, until all the parts function as a whole. More specifically, Erikson contends that there are eight psychosocial stages in the human life cycle. Each of these stages has a specific growth requirement, informed by a particular conflict, generated from the contention of instinctual and social demands on the person. Because of the urgency for successfully handling the developmental task for healthy maturation, each of these stages is a potential arena for crisis. If the specific developmental task that dominates that period of the life cycle is not successfully addressed, the person's ability to adapt will be adversely compromised by increased vulnerability to instinctual or social demands.

From the time of his classic, *Childhood and Society* (1950), until the 1980s (Erikson, 1982), Erikson left the decades between the twenties and the forties theoretically uncharted. Two major long-term studies of the lives of adult men have made decisive contributions to our understanding of the development of maturity during the intervening years. The first was conducted by George Valliant and his associates (1977). His study of men was concerned with determining which psychological mechanisms of defense are the most conducive to an adult life of satisfaction and well-being. Valliant's investigation empirically supported Erikson's hypothesis that the stages of the life cycle had the same sequence for each of the men studied and that no one stage was more vital than any other. Valliant's case histories suggested that men with mature defenses were far better equipped to love and to work than were those with more primitive defenses. More than half of the men found to have immature defenses were also suffering from serious emotional disorders. Furthermore, the employment of immature defenses was shown to precede rather than to follow the development of chronic physical illness. All of the men who at forty-five evinced mature psychological defenses continued to enjoy good physical health at fifty-five. They also were enjoying good friendships (Valliant, 1977).

The second important study of adult men's lives was conducted by Daniel Levinson and his associates (1978). Levinson's work followed Erikson's and was considerably influenced by it. At the same time, his study produced points of contention with Erikson impressionistic theory. In studying the biographies of a cross-section of forty contemporary American men, Levinson concluded that Erikson's notion that a single developmental issue dominates each of the life stages does not accurately capture the complexity of the developmental requirements of adulthood. For example, Erikson gives primary importance to the issues of generativity versus stagnation as the central task of mid-life. Using a Jungian conceptual reference, Levinson found that there are four different individuations (which I will discuss later on) that need to be resolved and integrated at mid-life in order for the person to be able to experience satisfaction and well-being in his life structure.

By life structure Levinson et al. (1978) mean

> the underlying pattern or design of a person's life at a given time. . . . A man's life has many components: his occupation, his love relationships, his marriage and family, his relation to himself, his use of solitude, his roles in various social contexts— all the relationships with individuals, groups and institutions that have significance for him. (p. 41)

Levinson found that the life structure unfolded in a relatively orderly and similar sequence for all of the men studied. Using Jung's notion of personal journey, Levinson conceptualized the lives he studied as a trek through different seasons, each having a qualitatively distinctive experiential character. Each of the realms of the journey has approaches and exists; they consist of:

> . . . a series of alternating stable (structure-building) periods and transitional (structural-changing) periods. These periods shape the course of adult psychosocial development. (p. 49)

Each of the developmental subphases also has an epigenetically different function:

> The primary task of every stable period is to build a life structure: a man must make certain key choices, form a structure around them, and pursue his goals and values within this structure. (p. 49)

The transitional subphase has a converse function to that of the stable period. A transitional period:

> . . . terminates the existing life structure and creates the possibility for a new one. The primary tasks of every transitional period are to question and to reapprise the existing structure, to explore various possibilities for change in self and world, and to move toward commitment to the crucial choices that form the basis for a new structure in the ensuing stable period. (p. 49)

Since each period of development has distinctive features and requirements, let us look specifically at the tasks of mid-life, in order to help us understand what may be the crucial developmental concerns and dilemmas for the seasoned practitioner.

What Does It Mean to Be a Middle-Aged Person?

Levinson et al. (1978) remind us that middle-aged men hope that life begins at forty. It is their great fear, however, that it actually ends there. This, I believe, is because by mid-life most men become acutely aware that *this is their real life*—it is not a dress rehearsal for some other stage of existence. The sense of being in the throes of real life comes from awareness of painful losses in our life and the prospect of a rapidly increasing departure of people whom we have known intimately, as well as diminishment of personal qualities that constituted integral parts of our sense of who we are.

Gould (1978) believes that the major false assumption of mid-life is that "there is no evil or death in the world." As with all other illusions, when we free ourselves from its deceptive security we find that the vulnerability it exposes in us has life-affirming potential, as well as its casting of anxiety about our capacity to take care of ourselves. Gould points out that liberation from the fallacies of youth

> . . . gives us access to the deepest strata of our minds that we have ever examined. It's our final natural opportunity to deal with the deeply buried sense of our "demonic badness" or "worthlessness" that has curtailed us from living as legitimate, authentic creatures with a full set of rights and a fully independent adult consciousness. (p. 293)

According to Levinson et al. (1978), still another fallacy to confront is the assumption that our failures and misfortunes have been imposed upon us rather than emanating from our own character. Consequently, in order to ably explore our yet untapped human potential, we first need to resolve the conflicts of our youth. In this crucial endeavor of mid-life and beyond, according to Gould's (1978) clinical assessment of male adulthood, we must

> . . . abandon old conspiracies, overcome remaining internal prohibitions and correct whatever distortions, misperceptions and misunderstandings that have prevented us from becoming authentic, whole people. (p. 293)

To do this, Levinson et al. (1978) indicate, a man must come to terms with the suppressed aspects of his character in terms of "the polarities that animate and divide him" (p. 245). At age forty or thereabouts, we are capable of doing this, because

> a man can make some judgments regarding his relative success or failure in meeting goals he set for himself in the enterprise of Becoming One's Own Man. . . . When a man experiences a developmental crisis in his late thirties, it stems from the overwhelming feeling that he cannot accomplish the tasks of Becoming One's Own Man. . . . (Levinson et al., 1978, p. 191)

A man who is confronted with the recognition that he has not fulfilled his cherished expectations of youth will be caught up in an identity crisis. Psychological novelists have long recognized wisdoms that we as psychologists have only recently incorporated into our developmental theories of adulthood. One of the most important of these is that life appears differently to the same person at different ages (Valliant, 1977).

One of the major causes of identity turmoil at mid-life has to do with the content of our earlier *dreams* of what our adult lives would be like. It is our youthful dreams, of course, that give our adult experiences their particular meaning. We do not live well in the climate of cold reality without the warm excitement of youthful dreams. We have to dream in order to survive. This is no less true spiritually and psychologically, than it is in terms of REM sleep. It is at mid-life that we are required by our epigenetic makeup to return to our childhood and adolescent dreams and carefully review what we believed our lives would be like as adults. Our happiness and optimism, as well as our despair and pessimism, are products of the quality of our sense of personal competence and well-being. We continually evaluate our competence and well-being subliminally in terms of how well we have fulfilled or even improved on our youthful dreams.

It follows that a frank exploration of the reasons why our dreams have not been fulfilled is vital in order to make realistic changes in our lives. Levinson et al.'s (1978) long-term research on the developmental stages in adult men's lives indicates that candidly examining our youthful dreams reveals three necessary tasks that must be worked on in passing from young adulthood to mid-life. They are:

1. We have to review and evaluate what we have done with our early adulthood.
2. We have to take initial steps to modify the unattainable and untoward strivings of our youth.
3. We have to deal with the polarities in our character that are sources of serious antagonisms in our relationship to ourselves, as well as with others.

Instead of courageously and diligently applying ourselves to the tasks of mid-life, we may become depressed and resolve to never again aspire and dream for anything beyond our ready reach. Or, manically, we may try to accomplish the complete fulfillment of our dreams in as short a time as we can. In short, not willing to confront our dreams, we may get caught up in desperate reactionary mechanisms, despite our knowledge as clinicians that these unwitting strategies will not give us a lasting sense of satisfaction and well-being.

Modifying the Dream

Of course, not all aspects of our youthful dreams are of equal importance. Some are more crucial than are others. Levinson tells us that for a man to derive a sense of satisfaction and well-being at mid-life, he must foremost modify what he dreamt it meant to become his own man. According to Levinson et al. (1978):

> The Dream thus contains an imagined self having a variety of goals, aspirations and values, conscious as well as unconscious, and pursuing his quest within a certain kind of world. A man's Dream is his personal myth, an imagined drama in which he is the central character, a would-be hero engaged in a noble quest. . . . (p. 245)

In examining what his dream has purported about what it means to become his own man, he will discover how much of it was based on illusions. Levinson et al. (1978) indicate that:

> Like most profoundly good things, the Dream is a mixed blessing. Certain aspects are conscious and tied to reality. But others are less conscious, less rational and more illusory. . . . The illusory aspects of the Dream become evident during the course of the Mid-Life Transition, [such as] the illusion of omniscience. . . . Jung speaks of "ego inflation," when a man experiences his internal hero figure as all powerful . . . the sense of omnipotence and the heroic drama give the Dream its intensity and its inspiration. But they contribute also to the tyranny of the Dream. Reducing the tyranny of the Dream is the major task of the Mid-Life transition. . . . (p. 246)

The dream contains an "if only" fallacy; therefore, to reach maturity a man is faced with the task of *de-illusionment*, in which he reappraises his values and goals, setting for himself realistic and flexible goals in terms of the person he is finally recognizing himself to be. In this crucial modification of his personal identity, Levinson et al. (1978) tell us, a person is faced with working on the *polarities* of his existence that need to be integrated in order to become a more realistic version of "his own man." According to Levinson, there are four polarities that need to be reconciliated at mid-life: (1) young/old; (2) destruction/creation; (3) masculine/feminine; (4) attachment/separation. Since these conflicting psychological tendencies exist throughout the entire life cycle and can never be resolutely done with, each developmental period in our lives gives us a fresh opportunity for their integration.

FEMALE ADULT DEVELOPMENT

Levinson (1978) chose to study only males in his important study of adult development because he believed that his findings about men could be generalized to women. He claimed that women go through the same developmental phases as men, although due to differences of biology and social values they experience these phases somewhat differently. Until recently the authors of major theories of human development have been men who shared Levinson's belief (Belenky et al., 1986). And because traditionally the subjects of research studies in psychology have been predominantly males, opportunity to empirically challenge the theorists' male bias has been limited (Gilligan, 1979). This can be confirmed by Erikson's eight stage theory. Although Erikson (1968) reports that adolescent girls don't deal with the identity crisis of "industry versus inferiority" as adolescent boys do, his conceptual scheme presents adolescence for boys and girls as if it did (Gilligan, 1982). These theories have crucial consequences for how women are regarded. To the extent that a woman's behavior deviates from how males are seen to mature, that woman is likely to be regarded as pathological or deficient (rather than the theory as inadequate).

In the last decade or so, several female theorists have provided theories of adult development, based in part on empirical evidence, that advance the thesis that women develop differently from men. There is a striking theoretical contrast between normal female development as conceptualized by female theorists and male development as described by Levinson et al. (1978). According to Levinson, the impetus for male growth derives from an effort to fulfill one's dream. This achievement is accomplished by "becoming one's own man"— achieving task mastery in one's work and successfully separating from one's mentor. In contrast, for women identity is defined by the ability to care for others, and mature growth is based on linkage rather than detachment, with value placed on interdependence and continued relationship (Sekaran and Hall, 1989).

Bardwick (1980) has developed the most comprehensive theory of female adult development at the present time. She sees the major differences in the male and female stages of development as occurring in the thirties and forties. Sekaran and Hall (1989) have summed up Bardwick's conceptualization of these age periods as follows:

> *Age 28–39: the age-thirty transition and the settling-down period of the second adult life structure.* This period represents a major gender difference. First, women now in their thirties have probably experienced a more profound and prolonged transition than men at the same age (and thus are out of sync with men) because of the effects of factors such as the "biological clock time," the effects of growing families, the values of the women's movement, and the continuing effects of traditional values. This cohort is a *transitional* one in many ways, pulled between two quite different generations. . . . Women at this age experience strong career changes, whether they are just establishing a career or in mid-career, as well as strong life and family changes.
>
> *Age 40–50: the mid-life transition and middle adulthood.* At this point women are feeling more secure and settled in their relationships and are moving towards more autonomy. Men are moving in just the opposite direction; as career and task demands diminish, they are able to become more sensitive to interpersonal relationships and to their internal psychological needs. Each gender is moving toward greater balance of autonomy and interdependence, but from different directions.

ACHIEVING WISDOM

Adult development generally has been explored in one of two ways. The notion that there are specific sequences of age-related developmental tasks, transitions, and critical periods is a recent theoretical conception (Gallos, 1989), although philosophers and poets intuitively have expressed this idea for centuries.

A theoretically more venerable approach to human development is the delineation of the stages of development necessary for the achievement of wisdom and maturity. Wisdom, as I discussed earlier, has always been identified as a positive benefit of aging. The most profound influences on contemporary Western society come from two great traditions — Ancient Greek (Western) philosophy and Eastern philosophy.

Western philosophy is the endeavor that conveys knowledge about the nature of the world based upon the requirements of logical and rational thinking. *Logical thinking* is reasoning that follows from its premises. *Rationality* is based on the idea that we can best predict the course of events by first observing prior events, seizing upon certain patterns and similarities contained in each of these events in contrast to all other events, and as a result classifying these purveyed events into distinct categories. Therefore, the unifying theme in Western philosophy derives from the premise that we can master our existence by interpreting the laws of nature by logical and rational thinking. Having mastered the laws of nature we can then control and direct nature by anticipating (predicting) the lawful actions of animate and inanimate objects (Goldberg, 1980). The person who best achieves wisdom, from the Western perspective, is one who is curious and inquisitive. Such a person investigates, probes, and seeks out answers about the mystery of nature and is never satisfied until he or she obtains an understanding sufficient to know what is best for that person.

In contrast, Eastern thought is based upon the premise that each of us is nature and therefore cannot stand apart from nature in such a way as to objectively observe its laws. In Eastern philosophy each of us is exhorted to act with or, perhaps more properly stated, *from within* nature. As such, control and prediction are neither useful or possible. Each of us comes to know the world by the unfolding of the world within ourselves (Goldberg, 1980). The wise person, from the perspective of Eastern philosophy, is one who has developed the meaning of life from direct, experiential knowledge of oneself. Unlike the Western prototype, this is not a person who has done much logical and rational reasoning about life. The wise individual evidences wisdom not by telling others what the ultimate nature of reality is but by teaching people how to experience it for themselves (Clayton and Birren, 1980). To make this wisdom possible, *compassion* and *orienting one's life around others* are necessary.

It is instructive to examine how enlightened mentors have helped their disciples become authentically transformed. Karl Jaspers' (1957) important study of paradigmatic figures in history is rather insightful in this matter. Jaspers tells us of the persons he studied — Socrates, Buddha, Confucius and Jesus — that their basic masculine character was natural and striking. Each of these mentors, although speaking in parables and dialectical contradictions, presented himself as ordinary, not as a special being. Each was concerned with the development of selfhood. They guided their disciples in examining their lives but resisted leading them into social action. They appeared not to regard their mission as telling their followers how to live their lives. Instead, they patiently demonstrated by personal example and fostered a climate in which their disciples could question for themselves how they conducted their lives — permitting them to come to their own conclusions. Above all, Jaspers demonstrates, these paradigmatic people did not teach their disciples to hate or sanction flight from those who oppose them. Their human love was unlimited and universal. Thus, to extrapolate to our day, although he may feel fear and doubt or resolute enlightenment during crises in his own professional career, the enabling mentor never cajoles his or her disciples to validate the mentor's beliefs or to do what the mentor will not. The true mentor does not need this dubious proof. By not presenting him/herself as all knowing and all powerful, the mentor gives the power of transformation to his/her disciples. By permitting them to become transformed by their own chosen ordeal rather than those he/she requires of them, the mentor permits them to become as wise as he/she. In contrast, the false prophets, as Jaspers regarded them, were leaders who manipulated reality. They persuaded by the force of their personality rather than encouraged their disciples to find their own inner convictions. The implications of these notions are examined in Chapter 10.

A recent theoretical account of the stage approach to delineating wisdom and maturity is found in the work of Donald Heath. Heath, a professor of psychology at Haverford College in Pennsylvania, has since the 1950s been charting the lives of men who were his students as undergraduates at Haverford College. When these men married or moved in with a woman, Heath followed the lives of these women as well. In this very extensive study, which is oddly little known considering that it is one of the longest studies on adult development ever carried out, Heath has visited and spent several days each decade in the homes of these men and women. Heath (1991) has drawn a number of conclusions about the qualities of personality that have been necessary for his subjects to lead healthy and satisfying adult lives. We will use some of his statements about maturity when we explore whether seasoned practitioners, by virtue of their extensive experience in examining the psyche, derive any personal benefits with regard to their own maturity.

Heath has operationally defined *maturity* as those indices that are key in predicting who will marry happily, feel fulfilled vocationally, and act virtuously. He has concluded from his four decades of research that men and women do not differ in how they develop maturity. In Heath's (1991) study, mature men and women were characterized by the following qualities:

1. are extraordinarily involved and busy people;
2. have androgynous capacities (especially female interpersonal skills);
3. have the ability to accurately self-reflect about their own psychological processes;
4. are highly sensitive to how they are relating to others;
5. are aware of their own values;
6. have developed a progressive understanding of how they have become the people they are;
7. have moved from self- to other-centeredness;
8. are involved in caring interpersonal relationships;
9. are developing progressively more humane values;
10. have universal frames of reference which enable them to identify empathically with diverse people;
11. have personality processes that are stable and resilient;
12. have interpersonal relationships that are selective, cooperative, and enduring;
13. have values underscored by courage and commitment;
14. are developing a self-concept which is increasingly stronger and more autonomous;
15. are genuine, spontaneous and natural;
16. have values which are consistently ordered so that success in one role is related to success in other roles.

In Chapter 8, I will critique the adult developmental theories I have discussed in this chapter, using this critique to indicate the requirements for a comprehensive theory of adult development.

— seven —

INTERVIEWS WITH TWELVE
PROMINENT ANALYSTS

My lifelong theme has been one of triumph over disaster.

—Dr. T.

There has to be a distinction made between those who are seasoned practitioners simply by virtue of their many years of clinical experience and those who are regarded as *masters* at their psychotherapeutic trade. What is a "master" practitioner? Two of the questionnaire respondents defined the master therapist in such a way that their combined definitions quite comprehensively describe the exceptional practitioner. I will use these descriptions as the operational definition of what is meant by master practitioner in this chapter.

"Master practitioners," said one questionnaire respondent, "have a thorough indoctrination in the theories and techniques of what they do, recognize the limitations of these theories and techniques, and know that each individual has the potential for having an entirely separate experience and a legitimately different way of looking at the world." Said the other questionnaire respondent, a master practitioner is "one who has brought his/her training, sensitivity, perceptiveness, compassion, intelligence and motivation to the clinical work and has shaped these resources and skills so that they are no longer 'techniques,' but rather an integral part of the therapist."

The practitioners whom I visited and interviewed were all recommended as exceptional practitioners by other experienced therapists whose judgment I respect. Thirty-four practitioners were recommended. Letters were sent to most. A few whom I knew rather well were telephoned. Twelve wrote back or called me and agreed to be interviewed. As a group, these twelve eminent practitioners were even more experienced than were the senior therapists who answered the questionnaire. They averaged about thirty-five years of clinical experience.

In this chapter I examine the psychological and social factors that the twelve eminent practitioners whom I interviewed revealed to me to be important in living and practicing fully and well. The material presented here, based on more than thirty hours of interviewing, is necessarily *selective*. Some of those interviewed speak more frequently in the following pages than do others. This is not to ignore or to slight any of these astute practitioners. It simply is a statement that in my opinion some of them, by their words and how they presented themselves, spoke more articulately about the issues being pursued in my study than did others.

The issues which are explored in this chapter are found in the Appendix. The interviews were efforts to tap a fuller account of the lives and practices of seasoned practitioners than was feasible by questionnaire alone. Moreover, comparing the interview information with the data generated by the questionnaires may give us some insight into why some senior practitioners thrive while others become disillusioned. However, it also should be acknowledged that direct comparisons between the interviewed therapists and those who provided information by questionnaire cannot give us an unequivocal understanding about how exceptional practitioners differ from their colleagues. Although those who answered the questionnaire were not specifically recommended to me during this study as exceptional practitioners who should be interviewed, this in no way suggests that many of them are not as skilled as those interviewed.

In interviewing these seasoned practitioners I was less interested in their theoretical explanations of why they practiced as they did than in their felt experiences about how one matures wisely and compassionately. It should be emphasized that a tape recorder was visible throughout each of the interviews. Clearly, some were more willing to talk candidly about personal feelings than were others.

That there were considerable differences among these senior practitioners about the significance of some of the factors that enable one to live and practice fully and well will not, I imagine, come as any surprise to the reader. At the end of the chapter conclusions will be drawn about my assessment of the salient qualities and experiences embodied by these eminent practitioners. The chapters to follow examine the question of whether being a seasoned practitioner is significantly related to acquiring mature wisdom.

THE INTERVIEWS

Dr. V.

Dr. V. is the most senior of those interviewed. He is in his late seventies and has over fifty years experience as a psychoanalytic practitioner. He is world renown as a clinical and psychometric researcher and the author of numerous books and articles.

My impression of Dr. V. is of a man who in senior maturity is physically vital and intellectually curious. As a younger man he was an accomplished athlete, and he is still physically active and robust. Yet, I sensed that, despite his enormous professional accomplishments, he is still not certain that he has proven himself. He frequently referred to his publications when he seemed to feel that he was not being understood in the interview. A strong theme in his discussion of his life and career was his perception that at certain important moments in his career he was an outsider and unacceptable to the establishment. In the German university in which he studied he experienced threats from fellow students and faculty who were members of the National Socialist Party. He also spoke of being ostracized for his research interests by the psychoanalytic establishment in this country. Although he was intellectually drawn to psychometric research, he sought a medical education and clinical training because as a physician he felt that he had a better chance to survive against the Nazis. They, he believed, were more apt to regard him as valuable as a physician than as a psychologist.

The most vibrant continual theme emerging from my interview with Dr. V. was that of his trying and usually succeeding to overcome adversity in his life by attending to latent and underdeveloped aspects of himself. The confluences of clinical practice with intellectual research curiosity and of physical development with intellectual prowess are two manifestations of this to which I have already alluded.

Dr. W.

Dr. W. is a psychoanalyst in his late forties who expresses his ideas articulately and enthusiastically. I saw none of the cant and the cynicism that a couple of the more senior practitioners exhibited during their interviews. I found that I had much in common with Dr. W., because both of us devote much of our professional life to writing and teaching. We also share the belief that our majoring in philosophy as undergraduates has been significant in our development as psychotherapists.

Dr. W. spoke of his being drawn to psychology and psychoanalysis from his experiences as a college student in analysis with someone with whom he could speak with freely. From these interactions he felt he gained some control over his life and formulated meaningful options for what to do with his future. His analyst, he told me, was unlike the angry and critical father with whom he grew up. In looking back he realizes that he has pursued the career of an analyst so that other people would feel about him as he did about his first analyst. He discussed how as a younger person he craved intimacy but, because of earlier painful experiences, needed to control the degree of closeness in his relationships.

His first analyst had not challenged his social withdrawal, permitting him overly protective distance. So when he became a therapist himself, he was threatened to find that many of his patients did not have any respect for his authority or for his privacy, and as a result violated his personhood in ways that were painful to him. His subsequent analyst was an improvement over the first in that this analyst enabled him to work out his interpersonal fears.

He indicated that, had he remained as distant as he had initially been, the work of psychoanalysis would soon have become tedious. Much of his personal development as a person and as an analyst has come from recovering from the initial shock of patients' intruding into his personal space. Important in the satisfaction he enjoys as a mature analyst is having overcome limitations in his character structure. He spoke of this process in terms of a dialectic development in his theoretical and clinical work. This point of view, crucial to my own notions about adult development, is discussed in the next chapter.

Dr. X.

Dr. X. is a mild, gentle man in his late seventies. A clinical psychology pioneer and the founder of a well-regarded psychoanalytic training program, he speaks about his career in rather modest terms, preferring to emphasize how fortunate he has been to have known and worked with brilliant and creative colleagues and students. He disclosed little about his personal feelings and his family life.

The dominant theme in Dr. X.'s interview, conducted in his institute office, was his deep regret about the loss of his intellectual and

vital capacities, which have forced him to give up practicing psychoanalysis. He has in recent years suffered several serious physical ill-
nesses. He apologized several times for his severe memory loss, saying
that he doesn't remember many of the details of his early career.

Dr. P.

Dr. P. is a gracious and active woman in her eighties who is still a
much sought after supervisor. She was one of the first psychologists
(and a woman psychologist at that) to practice psychoanalysis in the
United States. She was trained by psychiatrists who, fearing censure
by the medical establishment, trained her and two other women psychologists clandestinely. Dr. P. also was the first woman practitioner
to be the president of her interdisciplinary professional association.

The dominant theme in Dr. P.'s interview was her belief in the
power of a good training analysis to ably fortify the practitioner for
whatever vicissitudes of fortune may emerge at some time or other in
his or her practice. What she regards as a proper analysis is one that
adequately analyzes the analysand's preoedipal issues. She maintains
that those who experience serious conflicts in their analytic careers
undoubtedly have had their preoedipal conflicts unattended. She believes that there are few gender differences in the developmental issues
of male and female practitioners. In her view, what separates women
from men therapists is that married women are more likely to practice
part-time than married men. The quality of one's training analysis,
she maintains, is what distinguishes one analyst from another, regardless of gender.

Dr. Z.

Dr. Z. is a much sought after supervisor and teacher in his early
seventies. Because I have known him for many years, I know that he
is abundantly enjoyed as a witty and piquant story-teller as well.
What has always impressed me about him is his blending of blunt and
forceful straight talk with a considerable capacity for demonstrative
tenderness and sentimentality. I observed during the time I spent with
him that his personal identity is as readily conveyed by how he carries
himself as by his words. In addition to interviewing him in his home
office, I had the fortunate opportunity to be with him as he inter-
acted with friends and family at lunch.

The central theme in Dr. Z.'s interview, as with many of the other
practitioners interviewed, is the importance of having arrived at being a psychotherapist as a means of overcoming the negativity and

adversity of one's tender years. Dr. Z. said, "Whatever ability to do this work I have didn't come from graduate training but from my family—particularly my father, who had the talent to be a leader of men." This proclivity for psychological understanding was fostered in the painful crucible of his deep need to understand the disturbed family in which he grew up and in which he "was assigned the role in the family of getting educated to lead the savages [the other family members] out of the jungle."

Dr. Y.

Dr. Y. is a colleague in his early seventies whom I have known for many years. I was involved in two weekend-long training experiences led by him early in my career. He is regarded as a gentle and energetic analyst; many psychiatrists I know have told me that he provided the best training experience of their psychiatric residency.

While we sat in the lobby of the hotel where I was to give a presentation, Dr. Y. told me that he grew up feeling alien in a gentile culture. He came to the United States to get a certificate in education and then to return to Canada. While he was in college, a classmate gave him a book by Sigmund Freud. In reading the work he felt that Freud was speaking directly to him about his own questions about his Jewish identity.

The dominant theme in Dr. Y.'s interview is the all-consuming obsession being a practitioner and a teacher is for him. He reports that it colors most corners of his life. Together with being a practitioner, his greatest joy is to supervise and mentor young psychiatric residents. Continuing to teach, he said, has compensated him, replacing the losses in his life—his grown children who have left home and the colleagues who have retired or died. For Dr. Y., perhaps more so than some of the other senior practitioners interviewed, teaching and practicing seem to have such a strong definitional role in his personal identity that I wonder how he would define himself if his work were curtailed.

Dr. T.

Dr. T. is a warm and very enthusiastic European born analyst in her early fifties. Originally trained as a developmental psychologist, she has been strongly influenced by humanistic and existential psychology following her analytic training and has taken active leadership in the humanistic branch of psychology.

Of those interviewed, Dr. T. was one of the strongest advocates of the theme of triumph over adversity. A survivor of the Nazi holocaust, she said that her life has been bizarre, colored by the Second World War. To survive, her lifelong theme has been "my head is bloody but unbowed."

Dr. S.

Dr. S. is a Latin psychoanalyst in his early fifties and the director of a clinical psychology doctoral program. He has written extensively about cross-cultural psychology and psychotherapy. He has been a teaching colleague of mine for a number of years.

Dr. S. emphasized in his interview that master therapists develop over time a cognitive mind-set that enables them to conceptualize and understand patients (and themselves as well) in a more highly efficient way than they did as beginners. This ability to get quickly and accurately to the central fantasies and the life patterns people have created from these governing fantasies distinguishes the highly skilled seasoned practitioner from less experienced and mediocre practitioners.

Dr. A.

Dr. A. is a humanistically oriented practitioner originally trained as a social psychologist. She is highly regarded by other practitioners as knowledgeable and balanced in her views about the concerns that have come to be called "women's issues" in psychology. Although she has post-doctoral training in psychoanalytically oriented psychotherapy, she views her patients' issues less in terms of their intrapsychic dynamics than in terms of how they dispossess themselves of enabling interpersonal cooperative strategies for dealing with where they are in the world.

The dominant theme in Dr. A.'s interview was that psychotherapy practice is a metaphor for how the practitioner is in the world. Difficulties in the work itself, she claimed, should not be the focus of the practitioner's concern. Dr. A. pointed out that disappointment and disillusionment is inherent in life. No matter what career the troubled practitioner would have chosen, the problems probably would have been similar. Rather than be overly focused with the career aspects of the troubled therapist's life, it is wiser, she believes, for the practitioner to recognize how he or she understands the world and to deal with that world view.

Dr. Q.

Dr. Q. is a female practitioner in her mid-forties who was trained in a psychoanalytic post-doctoral training institute. She was recommended as a senior therapist who, while a highly skilled practitioner, puts her professional work into a balanced perspective with the other areas of her life.

The major theme in Dr. Q.'s interview is that her psychotherapy practice is only one important role in her life. She also is a wife, a mother and a caring friend to several special people in her life. There are times when roles other than being a psychotherapist have ascendancy in her priorities. If, for example, her child were ill, she would have no hesitation to leave her practice for as long as her child needed her. She reported that her close female friends who are psychotherapists share this attitude. In contrast, for the most part, she believes, being a psychotherapist is the overridingly important life role for the male practitioners she knows.

Dr. U.

Dr. U. is a very energetic and charismatic man in his mid seventies whose vitality gives him the appearance of a considerably younger man than he is. He has had over fifty years of clinical experience. Early in his career Dr. U. pioneered several innovative approaches to clinical practice and clinical research. His work has made important modifications in how patients and therapists work together and how they understand their therapeutic alliance. He has been the president of a number of large professional organizations.

The dominant theme in the interview was that, despite Levinson et al.'s (1978) claim that a man's adolescent dream is the compelling force that directs his vocational energies, neither he nor other practitioners he knows have had a definitive fantasy prior to becoming psychotherapists. He said that he stumbled into becoming a psychiatrist and psychoanalyst. Like so many of the others I interviewed, he recognizes that at least in the beginning his career was predicated on proving himself to be as worthy and competent as those who came from more privileged circumstances. In his case it was to prove that as a young doctor he was as good as the Harvard trained physicians he was competing against for medical positions during the Depression. The continual need to prove himself to be highly competent, he told me, has fostered an ongoing clinical depression.

Dr. R. — A Dissenting Perspective

I set aside for last my visit and interview with Dr. R. His views are rather discordant with those of the other master practitioners I interviewed.

Dr. R. is a renown training analyst and the author of several books on the cultural context of psychoanalysis. He is the director of one of the more prestigious psychoanalytic training institutes in the country. He was recommended to me by another very senior analyst as one of the smartest classmates in his analytic training institute, someone he would go to if he had a serious problem with a patient. I interviewed Dr. R. in his office close to this very same institute.

Dr. R. told me that his entering the field of psychiatry was quite undeliberate. Having a wide spectrum of interests, he could easily imagine being rather satisfied in a number of other careers. He entered college during the Depression. His father, who made a decent living as a physician, suggested that he, too, enter medicine. While in medical school he was primarily interested in neurology. He turned away from this medical subspecialty because he knew of only one neurologist in the city in which he trained who was able to make an adequate living in independent practice. Psychiatry residencies were easy to come by. And although he had not much of an idea about what psychiatry involved, he took a residency in psychiatry as a temporary measure, so that he would have some time to decide what he wanted to do with his medical training.

It was easy to slip into becoming a psychoanalyst in the early 1940s, he said. People were ashamed to seek out analytic treatment for personal reasons. Becoming an analyst, on the other hand, was a marvelous way of getting analyzed without embarrassment, obtaining training in a profession that seemed interesting and at the time was not inundated with practitioners. It also was prestigious enough to be the second highest paid medical subspecialty. When he entered his training analysis he thought of the analyst as a person who sits quietly in his chair, smokes his pipe, and enjoys some intriguing people revealing to him their most private feelings and fantasies.

Almost half a century later, Dr. R. has become increasingly disappointed by the loss of prestige of being an analyst, commenting that his less astute medical school classmates in other fields of medicine are making far more money than analysts do. Also, he has not found the work of the analyst to be the personally growthful experience he expected it to be when he entered the field and met analysts who acted as if they had found a special fount of wisdom.

I asked Dr. R. whether seasoned practitioners, as a result of their continuous examination of how other people live their lives, learn anything of practical value in living their own more maturely and wisely. He responded to me with a placid face, but his expressive hands conveyed a sense of exasperated disbelief at my misguided inquiry. As he turned his distinguished face, adorned with a full head of long, white hair, sideways, it seemed as if he wasn't sure whether to let me in on an important secret. While considering the matter, he removed some lint from his white silk shirt with a deft flick of his wrist. Finally, he paradoxically said to me:

> *At our institute candidates are soon dissuaded of any heroic myths they might have once harbored that their supervisors are particularly wise. Anyone who believes that there is a path to wisdom by being analyzed hasn't had a good training analysis.*

He went on to inform me that, while a personal analysis can be helpful in becoming a little more sensitized to one's own dynamics and participation in life, it serves little more. It certainly doesn't prepare one to live life better than someone who hasn't had an analysis.

Dr. R. paused again. His fingers caressed his cheek as he revealed a second important secret:

> *Analysis is a highly circumscribed game. It is played for particular purposes, such as becoming exquisitely attentive to oneself. It brings you a lot closer to the existential issues than people who haven't had an analysis. As a game, it works because it is an unreal situation, where you are protected from the stresses of living. So while it helps you understand psychological issues, it doesn't necessarily indicate what to do with this understanding. I know some people at seventy-five who have never been in analysis but who are quite effective, cheerful and happy. Are they any worse off for being less self-aware than the analyzed person who is depressed from what he has discovered about life from examining it closely?*

As Dr. R. spoke, I wondered where, in this day of scarce mental health dollars, he was able continually to fill a practice with people who weren't actually suffering and had the time and the money to amuse themselves with intriguing intellectual games. Evidently, his clinical practice is different from mine. Most of those I see suffer painfully from debilitating shame and despair. Several have made serious suicidal attempts. But I wondered if, in fact, Dr. R.'s patients could be that totally different from mine and those of the other practitioners I interviewed. Is it possible, I wondered, that he isn't completely honest with his patients? I could not easily suppress the thought that, although he regarded analysis as an intellectual game, which didn't effectively challenge the patient on how he or she related to society or enable the patient to reenter the world outside the consulting room with any discernible hope or skill in dealing with society, his patients were never informed of this. Perhaps, like Alan, the analyst in Chapter 2, Dr. R. thinks that patients should slowly discover for themselves that analysis is ill advised if they want to cope with issues that are painfully experienced as immediate and real.

But before I could pursue this line of inquiry, Dr. R., in startling vitriolic language that brought out a side of his personality that I had not experienced earlier, launched into providing evidence that analysts are frequently not helped by their analysis, training, or clinical experience. He virtually hissed:

All you have to do is to look at that collection of analysts who are social misfits, child molestors, and what not. And the rest of them don't have any better marriages than ordinary people either, nor are they better parents. Whether they are better prepared to handle aging and death than anyone else, I'm not certain. But I don't know of a single person who is an analyst who isn't afraid of dying.

Dr. R. was one of the last of the master practitioners I interviewed. Comparing his view of the existential meaning of the analyst's work with that of the others presented a considerable conceptual problem. Dr. R. is a highly regarded training analyst whose views cannot be readily dismissed. Yet his account of the function of analysis as a three- or four-times-a-week, five-year project that minutely examines one's entire being, but without any optimistic belief that the quality of that person's life would be improved by these considerable efforts, reminded me of a story of an unrealized child. This precocious child was skillfully able to take apart old clocks without breaking, bending, or losing a single part. However, he was entirely unable to put them together in such a way so that they would function to tell time. This disability didn't overly concern him, however. He, as a child with wealthy and indulgent parents, had his needs met as he experienced them. He didn't have to concern himself with structuring his life to meet others' needs.

In stark contrast to Dr. R., the other master practitioners seemed to believe that their psychic dispositions were such that they required continual psychological work on themselves in order to overcome earlier adversity. Being in a profession that daily examines the human psyche, they have come to realize a satisfying means of recasting unwanted aspects of themselves and, at the same time, acquiring some understanding of how a person's life may be lived fully and well.

In trying to understand why Dr. R. claims that psychoanalysis has minimal growth value for both patient and practitioner, let us consider first *the constancy fallacy* in regard to psychotherapeutic systems. Psychoanalysis does not exist as a generic entity. Yet Dr. R. and most other practitioners — in fact, most people — speak of psychoanalysis as if it were analogous to a routine medical procedure. In contrast to medical procedures, there are as many different psychotherapies as there are practitioners who conduct psychotherapy. This is the reason why it is so difficult to study "psychotherapy." Freud (1914) recognized this. He wrote:

> He who hopes to learn the fine art of the game of chess from books will soon discover that only the opening and closing moves of the game admit of exhaustive systematic description, and that the endless variety of the moves which develop from the opening defies description; the gap left in the instructions can only be filled in by the zealous study of games fought out by master-hands. The rules which can be laid down for the practical application of psychoanalysis in treatment are subject to similar limitations.

Freud (1912) recommended that each practitioner learn to conduct psychoanalysis in accordance with his own temperament and skills rather than assuming the analytic posture of some idealized practitioner conducting a standardized procedure.

When Dr. R. tells us that the specific kind of psychoanalysis *he practices* provides little to prepare his analysands to live well, I believe him. Who would know better than he that the way he conducts analysis is next to worthless for his patients in living more maturely? And who would be more qualified than he to ascertain that his experiences as an analyst and as a teacher have had little influence in living his own life any more wisely?

The second step in trying to understand why Dr. R. differs from the other eminent practitioners is to recognize that something important has not been explained by Dr. R. in his saying that his analysis doesn't enable people to live better. If Dr. R. offered nothing of value, why would his patients, many of whom are analysts and psychotherapists, have kept coming back to him?

For his therapist and analyst patients, the answer is obvious. He provides a role model for how to make an excellent livelihood as a practitioner. Beyond this I believe that Dr. R. does teach his patients something of life, but it is a highly *overcompromised* learning. What Dr. R. sells is learning to live as conflict-free as possible by viewing life *neutrally*, that is to say, without any great investment in the events in the world. This stance asks the individual who has been an analysand of his to respond to life as a series of questions that require only practical solutions. This point of view can be discerned from his response to my question about whether his view of neurosis and human nature have changed during his career. He answered:

> *I think that the most significant change in my view of neurosis is that when I began practicing psychoanalysis I had a profound contempt for patients. Even though I had gone through psychoanalysis, mine was a training analysis. I thought that there was something wrong with being a real patient. I believed for a long time that I was superior to my patients. But over the years I have come to realize that,* if you want to work effectively *with patients, the less you think about diagnostic categories and just* assume *that you are both ordinary people, the faster you will work. And it will be easier and more comfortable for you.*

What I believe is crucial about Dr. R.'s changed perspective is how he derived it. When asked whether his change of view was a natural consequence of his life experiences or clinical experience over the years, he covered his eyes with his palm for a moment. Composing himself, he informed me that he doesn't feel any wiser today than three decades ago when he was thirty-five. He emphasized that his clinical practices were based solely on his clinical experience and the practical cleverness of H. S. Sullivan, who had demonstrated "that we are all more similar than otherwise."

It is ironically revealing that Dr. R. quotes Harry Stack Sullivan as purporting to be an ordinary man. A brilliant intuitive clinician, Sullivan was a strange and most tortured man. He was said by his former associates to be able to speak about mental illness with the authority of one who was emotionally cold, detached, withdrawn, and fearful of intimacy (Ehrenwald, 1976). Given Sullivan's superior psychological insight, he could hardly have regarded himself as ordinary. Dr. R. is well aware of this. I came away from my visit with him with the impression that his statements reflect the disingenuousness of an analyst who is only pretending that he doesn't know everything about everything.

However, whatever Dr. R.'s hidden beliefs may be, they are not the focus of this book. I have given considerable attention to his views about the maturity of the practitioner because I suspect he represents a number of other bored senior practitioners. Fortunately, his perspective doesn't hold proxy for the other analysts interviewed. In the pages to follow I examine what the other senior practitioners said about the issues, concerns, and dilemmas of mature practice.

The Role of Mentor in Mature Practice

The study of the lives of creative and accomplished people reveals that mentors play a vital role in constructive human development. Like psychotherapists, they serve as psychological teachers in searching the psyche for ways to live one's life with purpose.

Dr. Y. had Elvin Semrad for a mentor for much of his career. He said that Semrad "had to be seen in the flesh to be believed. He taught by example. He was very absorbing. You don't see many of his type today. Actually, I've had very few good teachers along the way. That is why Semrad was so special to me."

Having had an inspired mentor stimulates the desire to teach and mentor others. Looking at the middle seasons of life, Erikson (1950) tells us the most important relationship a man will have develops from his *generativity* needs:

> Mature man needs to be needed, and maturity needs guidance as well as encouragement from what has been produced and must be taken care of. (pp. 266–267)

For the seasoned practitioner, being a mentor (or even a writer for that matter) fosters the Heisenberg principle—it changes in subtle ways how one practices. Most of the master practitioners interviewed spoke of teaching and serving as a mentor as invigorating a clinical practice that would soon grow stale without the continual challenges presented by students. Dr. W. pointed out that one's students (as does one's reading audience) take on the role of nonpresent observers of one's clinical work, stimulating a constructive inner dialogue about one's ideas and practices. For younger and less experienced practitioners, supervisors may play this nonpresent observer role as critical introjects.

These master practitioners, unlike a number of the seasoned practitioners who answered the questionnaire, were all fortunate to have had available to them mentors who were role-models of actualized people, emulating an effective model of interpersonal competence and self-mastery. At best, mentoring is a statement of non-intrusive caring. The psychotherapist demonstrates this capacity by encouraging the younger practitioner to believe in his own good intentions. Levinson et al. (1978) give us some idea of what this involves when they indicate that the importance of the mentor is "sharing the youthful dream, and giving it his blessing, helping to define the newly emerging self in its newly discovered world and creating a space in which the young man can work on a reasonably satisfactory life structure that contains the dream" (p. 99).

In terms of therapeutic supervision, the master practitioners indicated that from their own experiences, both as supervisees and as teachers, the best mentoring came from those supervisors who were willing to be there for their students rather than to figure out clinical problems for them. It was exemplified by listening responsively and making personal statements rather than taking the more convenient route and giving advice or making interpretations about the reasons for the younger practitioner's problem. When the apprentice therapist was in distress about his clinical work, the supervisor's primary concern was that the young practitioner's struggle to examine his assumptions about him or herself enable him/her to follow his own path toward self-definition as a therapist, rather than taking a route that the supervisor, the training director, or parental introjects wanted. Nietzsche (1887) exhorted the physician (he speaks to the teacher and mentor as well) not to reproduce one's own state of being in the person being counselled but to encourage something higher. To do this, those who guide others have to overcome the *Laius complex* that has contaminated untold numbers of father-son relationships throughout history—the fear of being surpassed by the younger generation.

Mentors who possessed the capacity to lay aside their Laiusian fears were, according to Dr. V., men who had lived full and active lives before becoming analysts. His mentors, Ernest Kris and Rene Spitz (who had been his analysts first), had rich life experiences from which to hear and make sense of the longings of those they guided.

In the final analysis, the enabling psychotherapy mentor is ultimately concerned with the development of the young practitioner's *humanity*. Dr. Y. spoke of his mentor, Elvin Semrad, responding to a psychiatric resident who asked him how he derived his capacity to help patients overcome their losses, loneliness, and despair. Semrad was said to reply:

> It comes from a life of sorrow, and the opportunity that some people give me to overcome it and deal with it. The patient is the only textbook that we will ever need.

These considerations may help us see that psychotherapy training without competent and wise mentoring is generally deficient. In formal training programs we give considerable attention to intrapsychic impediments to interpersonal relations, as well as abundant amounts of technological knowledge in understanding clients and being able to maintain a relationship with them (Goldberg, 1976). At the same time, we provide no training in how to utilize best our own life experiences. Several of the eminent practitioners who tell their stories in Burton's 1972 book expressed considerable disappointment in their teachers, even those who were famous in the field. O. S. English wrote:

> . . . I cannot recall that I learned anything whatever from psychoanalytic supervisors. . . . not one of them ever said anything or commented on the work reported in a way that has remained with me. . . . I have often wondered why such great names in the field seem to mean so little in my training when I can still recall the helpful impact of many an unpretentious clinic patient. (Burton, 1972, p. 93)

In essence, the psychotherapist mentor gives the neophyte practitioner a sense of what the career of psychotherapist (from the special vantage of the examiner of the human psyche) can offer in living life more fully.

THE PERILS OF PRACTICE

Like the questionnaire respondents, several of the master practitioners identified the problem of *intimacy* as core to the dilemmas of clinical practice. Of course, therapeutic intimacy differs from intimacy experienced in everyday life. *Therapeutic intimacy* has a *time*, a *place*, and the imposition of *explicit comment* upon the processes and dynamics of its ongoing encounters in the consulting room.

These three components are required to differentiate therapeutic intimacy from its more commonplace expression, because the bond between therapist and patient is not of love—rather, we might say that love is not required—but of desire for shared discovery.

The striving for therapeutic intimacy emanates from an accentuated sense of being held off from the other and a wish to bridge that separation. The hallmark of therapeutic strivings, in contrast to love, is an immediate encounter and exchange of intentionality, as the encounter reveals and articulates the meaning of these two individuals' being together. The act of love may intend toward the other, but not necessarily requires the articulation of what is felt. Because of the openness to the other that intimacy requires, protective guards dissipate, encouraging a fusion of self and other. Without the imposition of realistic limits upon the therapeutic relationship, the patient can expect—indeed demand—that all his or her immediate needs be met by the therapeutic relationship.

One practitioner wrote on his questionnaire that the establishment of intimacy is one of life's most difficult tasks. But, he added, many practitioners "blame interpersonal disruptions on the psychopathology of the patient rather than recognize the difficulty of the task and help individuals to view the difficulties in a positive way." For practitioners with intimacy problems, said Dr. W., being constricted is a defense against being left alone with another person in a basically open-ended situation. Getting tired of therapeutic work, said Dr. Z., may be a way of denying the despair of being alone with another person and not being able to deal with the closeness. This is reflected in a published statement of two senior practitioners, who wrote that the fatigue of practice is due to the work taking such a long while, "particularly if the therapist does psychoanalytic work [and] sees the same people much of the time . . . " (Welt and Herron, 1990, p. 38).

Exacting work with relatively few people may result in considerably more *isolation* for the senior practitioner than for the beginner. The younger practitioner usually works with others—in a clinic, a hospital, or a group practice. All those whom I interviewed were in solo practices and have been for many years. There often is considerable *disillusionment* that accompanies solitary clinical practice. Many practitioners don't like self-employment. All of the senior practitioners interviewed spoke of dislike for at least some aspects of the business side of practice. As beginners they had to work hard at promoting their practice and gaining an efficient network. One psychologist, Dr. Z., had considered going back to school to gain a medical degree solely for business considerations.

In the past, the seasoned practitioner could easily maintain as large a practice as he wished. Most of his referrals sought long-term treatment and some prospective patients had to wait many months to be seen by very eminent practitioners. Many seasoned practitioners did not afford themselves much breathing room in scheduling their practices. This is no longer true. In recent years there has been a considerable change in the public's interest in psychological services. The practitioners interviewed, because of their esteemed reputations, have not yet actually suffered from a lack of filled clinical hours. A couple, because of their age, have considered cutting down their clinical hours. But all spoke of a recent phenomenon for eminent, seasoned analysts who for years have had filled practices — the anxiety that they may never again see a real analytic patient and that they will be like every other practitioner, anxiously seeking to fill their practice with any referral they can get. Said Dr. U., "I was lucky. I came into the field at the right time. Now is not the right time. It isn't that I am disillusioned about doing psychotherapy and psychoanalysis. I love it. It is just that the phone doesn't ring much anymore."

According to Dr. X., who directs a large postdoctoral training program, because of the shortage of therapy patients, many senior practitioners hold onto patients longer than they should. This clinical educator pointed out several other perils of solitary practice. He spoke of the *intensity of the countertransference* for even seasoned practitioners. He indicated that when they begin their career therapists don't anticipate the strong attractions they will have toward patients, especially at times of crisis and vulnerability in their lives, such as significant losses in their private lives. As a result, there is much more sexual acting out than any of us would have imagined in the past, he said.

Senior therapists involved in inappropriate "acting out" are usually suffering from serious *disillusionment* about the career to which they have made a deep personal commitment. Their inability to find meaning in their work and in their private lives, Dr. Y. indicated, often leads them to distractions such as grabs for power, sexual affairs, delusions of grandeur and superiority, as well as misuse of alcohol and drugs. These palliatives are attempts to mask their depression and despair. Moreover, the sexual impotence many of these disillusioned practitioners suffer from reflects the overall helplessness they experience in life. When I pointed out that a number of younger therapists, who have only been in the field a few years, seem to be "burnt out," unlike the practitioners one reads about from yesteryear, Dr. V. (who has well over seventy publications) indicated that he believes this is reflective of a general cultural pattern, not of psychotherapists alone. In their souls, neophyte practitioners don't realize how difficult therapeutic work really is. They initially think that they can play-act at being psychotherapists. I was told that people today are not used to working as hard as people did in the past, when they expected to put in a hard day's work every day. One analyst, close to seventy years of age, said, at least in part seriously, "I can only work now a sixty-hour week. But after that I'm not good for anything else. The body refuses to do more."

Another senior practitioner, Dr. Z., pointed out that there was a certain "spiritual" reason that psychoanalysts of yesteryear did not seem to show manifestations of being burnt out as quickly as today. "They were," I was told, "zealots and missionaries for a new religion for healing tortured souls and had the energy and drivenness of preachers of a new faith."*

All religions have their secular politics. Psychotherapy is no exception. Dr. Y. spoke disconcertingly about the vicious power struggles and politics that many senior practitioners are involved in to gain prestige and adulation from their colleagues. After all, it was pointed out by Dr. W., there are few tangible rewards that we can bestow on our colleagues. Certainly, psychotherapists receive nothing like the material rewards and recognition that performers and business people receive. In large part, the most important part of our professional lives, our clinical work, is usually unseen by our colleagues. Our work is more subjective and more difficult to communicate intelligibly to even our most astute peers than are other kinds of professional endeavor. Clinically, we really don't know how well we practice as compared to our peers. Even many seasoned practitioners are often not sure what parts of their work they can truly take pride in and what professional tasks could have been done as well by mediocre practitioners. This contributes to an attitude of "closet competition" which does not foster a cooperative attitude toward our colleagues.

---

*These early practitioners of psychoanalysis were fervent in their desire to learn the art of conducting an analysis. When they had difficulty attracting analytic patients, some even paid patients to be analyzed. Dr. R. told of a medical colleague of his uncle who needed clinical experience—although he was not affluent, he offered patients 50 cents an analytic session.

More than other professions, we struggle with our professional and personal issues alone. Perhaps there are analysts who go out to lunch together, Dr. V. reflected, but he did not personally know of any. His attorney patients, on the other hand, met colleagues regularly at the Yale Club for lunch. For practitioners hungry for recognition, professional politics serves as a powerful avenue for prestige.

The Effect of Aging and Problems With Health

One of the more senior practitioners, Dr. X., told me that he had stopped practicing analysis due to the effects of aging. In recent years he had suffered some serious health problems. As analysts, he said, we have a long-term commitment to our patients. He found himself trying to hurry up the analysis because he didn't know how long he would be able to practice. He also experienced memory loss and a tendency to tire easily. There were other unfortunate side-effects. Patients who learned of his illness were especially careful not to express negative emotions in their sessions. This fostered an unacceptable inferior analytic situation.

The recognition of special problems in each of the stages of adult development suggests that we need to differentiate the concerns of the mid-life practitioner from those of senior maturity. Eissler (1977) has indicated that aging in the older practitioner may have a different effect on the practitioner's narcissism than it had earlier in his career. According to Eissler, the analyst's aging assumes one of the three major trends:

1. The practitioner will become rigid, intolerant and compulsive if concerns about the effects of the loss of his vitality are involved with his idealized sense of himself.
2. He will expect and demand admiration from his patients and respect from his colleagues if his concerns about lost analytic skills center on his ability to function as adequately when aged as he did earlier in his career.
3. Or he may show increased tolerance and acceptance of the limitations of his patients by sensing from his own difficulties the universality of human finitude.

The lessening of therapeutic ambition, Eissler maintains, frees the practitioner to concentrate on knowledge and understanding of the human condition rather than on desire that the patient make decisive changes in his life to satisfy the practitioner's therapeutic ambitions.

The specific concerns of each of the stages of the practitioner's life cycle has led Warkentin and Valerius (1975) to recommend that personal therapy continue as long as the therapist practices.

Practice may be influenced as much by one's social network as by one's person. Another veteran practitioner, Dr. Z., who had suffered serious illness indicated that his *own* illness was of little impediment to careful clinical work. What did affect his work, however, was the health of members of his family. In the course of long-term treatment, inevitably a problem will arise in one's own family. These were the moments in his clinical practice when he was more likely to be preoccupied and not at his best.

BURN-OUT

Is "burn-out" in the nature of the work we do or due to the kind of people we are? A study examining this question was conducted by a San Francisco psychiatrist, Bermak (1977), who surveyed 75 psychiatrists in the Bay area. The study strongly suggests that psychiatrists themselves believe that they have special emotional difficulties. The findings of this study were supported by all but two of the therapists I interviewed. Dr. A. seemed to believe that therapists have the same vocational issues as do others. Dr. Z. agreed by pointing out, "I think that those practitioners who burn out do so because of their own issues and would probably do so no matter what kind of work they did." On the other hand, Dr. W. indicated, "We probably have to be a little nuts to begin with in going into this business. I would imagine that as a group we are more than the average in a propensity for depression." Another, Dr. V., felt that there was an interaction between the stress of the work and the character of the practitioner, "Maybe we start out more isolated than other people, but the nature of the work reinforces the problem of feelings of pessimism about life."

This pessimism may be reflected in a lack of "generosity of spirit." Some senior practitioners, Dr. V. pointed out, don't show their patients the same sensitive consideration they show themselves in responding to pain and suffering. Analysis is a painful process that shouldn't be made any more difficult than it has to be. Dr. V. believes that there is too much emphasis placed on psychopathology in analytic work, using the metaphor of analysts often turning lice into elephants. He indicated that we too often forget that our patients may be highly competent and accomplished people outside of our consulting rooms.

MATURITY OF THE PRACTITIONER

Since the practitioners I interviewed are highly regarded by their colleagues, they should have a strong personal sense about what constitutes a *mature practitioner*. The most cogent statement on this issue was stated by Dr. Z., who indicated:

> *The mature practitioner should be a more effective therapist not be-*
> *cause he has more knowledge and expertise about the craft of psycho-*
> *therapy but because he has lived more fully and knows himself better*
> *than the younger therapist. If you are really mature in this business,*
> *then what you do is to become more and more who you are. At some*
> *point you stop trying to do therapy and you are just yourself with your*
> *patients — given the goals you and he have decided to pursue for that*
> *particular person.*

The confluence of the person of the practitioner and the way he practices was confirmed in the statement of a second analyst, Dr. U., a practitioner of almost five full decades. He said with considerable zeal:

> *If you are a therapist, you think and feel like a therapist wherever you*
> *are — when you are running in your sweat clothes, out at the pool in*
> *your bathing suit or even reading a magazine on the toilet. Being a*
> *mature analyst requires some common sense. Some analysts tend to*
> *get too caught up with technique and cannot as a result respond intelli-*
> *gently to everyday situations. They mistake the place (the couch) with*
> *the process. If Bernard Baruch could use a park bench in Central Park*
> *to conduct business, why can't I do therapy in the park or in the*
> *backyard of my house at the seashore!*

Two of the female practitioners interviewed, Drs. A. and Q., confirmed the common wisdom that women mature differently than do men. In general, they seem to accept aging better than do men; as a result, they are less caught up fighting or denying the physiological changes they are experiencing.

Some of the differences in maturity were attributed to value differences. Heath (1991) has indicated from his study of adults who live fully and well that they are capable of flexible androgynous functioning. In this regard, Dr. T., a humanistically oriented psychologist, believes that among therapists role functioning does not closely accord with traditional mores about gender. She feels that the qualities exhibited as a practitioner have more to do with professional discipline and value orientation than with whether one is a male or a female. Psychologists and social workers, she believes, tend to be more maternal, while psychiatrists are more paternal. Humanistically oriented therapists tend to play both paternal and maternal roles in their clinical work. A mature practitioner of either gender, she maintains, is androgynous.

Another important indication of therapeutic maturity, Dr. U. told me, is giving up "the myth of the hero." Most beginning practitioners feel the continual presence of concerned introjects scrutinizing their clinical work. Usually these are supervisors one admires, eminent practitioners one has met at professional meetings, or even master practitioners whose books one has read. Too often, in doing therapy the young practitioner may be responding more intently to what he believes are the expectations of his "observers" than to the needs of his patients. The young practitioner may imagine dialogues with his introjects in which he attempts to convince them of his skills as a therapist. "Maturity," said Dr. U., "is allowing the child in you to grow and mature. I couldn't start to be a decent analyst myself until I recognized that the 'cold bastard' I had as training analyst couldn't care less what kind of therapist I was. I had to do the best for me, not for someone else."

As a result of not being involved in defensive dialogue with critical introjects, Dr. S. indicated, the clinical work of the skilled mature practitioner is shortened and intensified. The therapist is less involved in the artifacts of therapy and more skilled at getting at what is significant than when he was a beginner. Consequently, the time spent is more therapeutically meaningful and its effects more lasting, even though he may be working less hard than when he was younger. The mature practitioner experiences time more preciously. He wants to get at the essence of things quickly and to use his time expediently. We see a parallel process of skillful clinical practice and mature life experience, when Dr. Q. indicates that the mature therapist with countless clinical experiences can say to a patient in crisis, "This shall also pass."

It may be appropriate, even necessary, for the young practitioner to take his time, rely more on theory, and not move decisively on clinical issues; on the other hand, the mature therapist compensates for the deleterious effects of aging with a sureness born of having visited many psychic lands before. Being older gives these therapists a freedom to say things without restraint. They don't need to beat around the bush. Their time is limited.

Maturity, no less importantly, also has an improved receptive quality. One practitioner, Dr. X., indicated that the mature therapist doesn't use his expertise to tell his patients how to live better; rather, he listens better than he did as a younger man from the context of his own life experiences. It isn't always a question of whether he is a *better* therapist than when he was younger. But he should be a *different* kind of practitioner. The younger therapist usually doesn't have the life experiences the older practitioner has and so must use his enthusiasm and his curiosity differently than the older, more tested practitioner. However, Dr. X. cautioned against assuming that those with the most stimulating life experiences are necessarily the most able therapists. "He might not be a very introspective and empathetic person. He also might be too active," said Dr. X. On the other hand, Dr. A. is a very active therapist. She said, "I just can't think about theoretical conceptualizations. I think of the person's issues in terms of the problem and the practical ways of dealing with it."

Life experiences themselves are not, of course, what matters; rather, what is key is what we do with them. Dr. Z. indicated that his beliefs about neurosis and human nature hadn't changed much over the years. But they have certainly softened. He said, "Now I don't see my patients as so different from me." Said another, Dr. Y.,

After thirty years of practice, I now see the positive side of psychopathology. I now see the meaning and value of disturbed behavior. Before I would shame the patient because of his neurosis. The first few years of practice I thought that everyone had to be like me. This wears you down after a while. You find out that people have to be who they are. It is a fallacious message, I believe, that you know how another person should live. I believe the message you want to convey is that I go about my life being the person who I am and I have come to terms with that person. In doing so I let my patients share my humanity and don't try to hide that I'm not perfect. But I am reasonably comfortable with myself. It is a freedom and a goal that they can recognize in being with me that they can achieve for themselves. As a therapist, I convey the belief that together we can find out who they are.

One of the best ways of teaching patients to trust themselves is by demonstrating our willingness to learn from them. To accomplish this we must carefully examine our presuppositions. Dr. V. told a humorous story of treating an actor patient who appeared to have a systematic delusion. He described his business agent as "stinking"; his wife, his children, his friends, and so forth, the same way. After a few months, it was necessary to see the wife. The analyst was startled upon meeting her to realize that the woman actually did smell. She was a schizophrenic and never bathed. Another analyst, Dr. Y., illustrated how he came to recognize the compensatory benefits of psychopathology in working with a very paranoid scientist. The patient never fully overcame his acute suspiciousness. However, treatment enabled the patient to turn his preoccupation with danger into ingenious methods of detecting and removing toxic materials from the atmosphere in his work as a chemist.

The seasoned practitioner also may harbor his own toxic material in the form of disguised feelings. He needs a reliable method of recognizing and treating these untoward feelings. In 1912 Freud expressed the opinion that every analyst should prepare himself for his difficult work by conducting his own self analysis. For Freud himself the examination of his dreams appeared to be the best method for scrutinizing the promptings of his psyche. He found it a very valuable psychological resource. Other introspective people have not been as skillful or courageous in their self-examination. Chessick (1977) points out quite accurately that, despite Socrates's intellectual brilliance in probing other men's innermost thoughts, he himself never appeared to recognize his own narcissistic intolerance of other people.

What did I learn about the self-examination of the eminent analysts whom I interviewed? Each of them reported self-analysis to be highly helpful. But, like the respondents on the questionnaire, few practiced it on a regular basis. Dr. Z. is typical in this regard. He told me:

I wouldn't call it "analyzing" but thinking about oneself and what one does. There is no question that it is helpful. But so is talking to Jesse, a friend and colleague for over thirty years, on at least a weekly basis. I have other sources of support and revitalization as well. On a monthly basis I meet with a small group of other senior analysts, all directors of training programs, and we discuss whatever the hell is going on in our private lives as well as in our practices, with the utmost candor.

Among the analysts interviewed, Dr. V. makes the strongest case for self-analysis. He has a unique method for his self-examination that he has found valuable for the past thirty years. He turns on a tape recorder and lies on his analytic couch and reports his dreams out loud. Then he reverses the analytic positions. He sits in the analyst's chair and listens afresh to the dreams that he has just recorded, examining them as he would a patient's material. He believes that in this way he is able to discern the hidden messages of unresolved issues that introspection alone would not reveal.

THE STATUS OF THE THEORY GUIDING THE INTERVIEWED PRACTITIONERS

In trying to understand how these master therapists differ from other experienced and more mediocre practitioners, it is useful to examine their approaches to psychoanalytic theory. They were unlike the questionnaire respondents, who, if they identified themselves as psychoanalytically trained, for the most part described psychoanalytic theory as either hopelessly flawed or beyond reproach. The master practitioners seemed to present the guiding theory for the way they work in much the same way that psychoanalysis was once regarded — as a radical and revolutionary force in society. Psychoanalysis in its early days represented for the most part a group of intellectuals with strong socialistic ideals and an accentuated artistic temperament. It is hardly surprising that in the early decades of the psychoanalytic movement in America a disproportionate number of analysts lived or practiced in Greenwich Village. When the movement became well-established and secured for the practitioner an affluent way of life, a migration from The Village to Park Avenue and the suburbs coincided (Jacoby, 1983).

The revolutionary force of psychoanalysis peaked in the 1960s and was replaced in that era by the Encounter and New group therapy movements (Goldberg, 1973). Clarence P. Oberndorf (1953), who was one of the earliest American psychoanalysts and had studied with Freud, wrote in his history of American psychoanalysis:

Psychoanalysis had finally become legitimate and respectable [and in so doing had paid] the price in becoming sluggish and smug, hence attractive to an increasing number of minds which find security in conformity and propriety. (p. 207)

With the exception of Dr. U. (and possibly Dr. R.), the master practitioners interviewed, unlike many of the practitioners who responded to the questionnaire, said that they had had good personal analyses. They referred to their former analysts with fondness and warmth. In turn, these master practitioners spoke of their guiding theory as a living language which grew out of their experiences in their own analysis and which is still open to experimentation based on their own personal experiences — even more than clinical events. Moreover, unlike so many of my other colleagues whose discussions of their clinical work is informed by the language of cant and psychodynamic "metatalk," the analysts interviewed spoke plainly, in everyday language. When they gave examples of their theoretical points, they as often provided themselves as existential illustrations.

Several have retained a radical, questioning fervor toward the psychoanalytic theory that guides their work. Some have taken what might be regarded as controversial positions. For example, Drs. A., U., and Z. have articulated the conviction that if psychotherapy is confined to the verbal dialogue of the analyst's consulting room its capacity to enlighten patients about crucial issues in their lives is inherently limited. Genuine healing, they maintain, requires the full presence of the therapeutic participants. Conventional analytic theory has maintained that this can occur by verbal disclosure and exchange alone. These three practitioners are among those critics of traditional analytic theory who have questioned whether words alone can reveal our authentic presence. Aren't our actions — as they underscore our values and especially those that contradict our verbal statements of intention — no less vital to be observed and experienced in authentically knowing the other? And if our actions are crucial in revealing who we are and enabling us to become who we intend to be, then isn't it egocentrically limited not to step out of the confines of the analytic hour and seek an arena in which the practitioner can encourage the patient's involvement in *social action* supportive of his or her emerging self-definition? Several of the analysts alluded to interactions with patients outside of the consulting room that were intended to have a therapeutic effect and to role-model appropriate interpersonal behavior.

What conclusions can be drawn from the reports of these articulate and thoughtful mature practitioners? There is a clear consensus that there is nothing any of them would rather do than practice psychoanalysis. All appeared to enjoy the emotional engagement of therapeutic work and, except for one, they felt optimistic that their work would continue to have a salubrious effect on the lives of those with whom they work. One of the youngest of these practitioners, Dr. W., said that, not only is he satisfied with practicing as an analyst, but he also finds himself more content as each year passes.

As a group they stood out in five basic ways:

1. There is in their personal and therapeutic mission a theme of overcoming adversity.
2. Their understanding of themselves and their patients is markedly characterized by their ability to relate theirs and their patients' particularistic concerns to a more universal vision of what is important in life.
3. Their maturity has a vital presence.
4. They show an ongoing curiosity about self and others that comes from a love of discovery.
5. They show strong oppositional forces in their personalities.

In the remaining chapters I will examine these salient features of the master therapists in terms of the larger context of adult development.

eight

Toward an Existential Theory of Human Development

> If there is an answer to the problem of meaning in my
> life, it does not lie out there someplace, but within me.
> Life does not present me with meaning. Life merely is.
> The meaning, the zest for living, comes from a full
> involvement with life.
>
> —H. F. Thomas, 1967

There is a tale told from ancient time about a lovely maiden whose greatest joy came from gazing upon herself in the reflection of her daily outdoor bath. One dark morning she peered at her bath water and discovered with horror that the figure she saw reflecting back at her had no head. She became panic-stricken and ran around shrieking, "My head is gone! Where is my head? Who has seen my head? I shall surely perish if I don't find my head!"

When her friends tried to reassure her that she still had her head on top of her neck, she refused to believe them. She hysterically insisted that every time she looked at her reflection her head was completely missing.

Suddenly, one of her more audacious friends gave her a sharp clout on top of her head. The maiden cried out in pain. Her clever friend informed her that, although the maiden had deluded herself into believing that her head was not available to her, she was nevertheless suffering from its presence.

So it is with our ability to make sense of our existence. We spend a lifetime asking questions concerning our personal identity: "Who am I?" "Where am I?" "Why am I?"

At various moments of our lives we have responded differently, depending on the degree of clarity present at those periods of our lives. And as we think back, we may recognize that the clarity of our perspective was not necessarily progressive. It was said of one well-known political journalist that he entered Yale University as an intellectually precocious freshman and graduated at about the same level of maturity. Our momentary clarity of perspective is proportional to the success we are having with the maturational issues of that current stage of life, no matter how brilliant and self-realized we may have been earlier in our lives. In this chapter I will present a theoretical rationale to account for why maturity, contrary to popular belief, is not always progressive.

ARE MID-LIFE PSYCHOTHERAPISTS LIKE OTHER PEOPLE?

In the past many people outside the field of psychotherapy have asked me whether psychotherapists are successful practitioners of their own art. I have answered that if they were then they would probably be unique among professionals. Experienced physicians are not necessarily healthier than the average person, attorneys as a group are not extraordinarily judicious in their private lives. But, of course, no one actually knows the answer to whether or not psychotherapists wisely utilize their knowledge in their lives, whether they live like other people or, on the other hand, use their professional stance to avoid the aspects of living that expose their vulnerabilities. No one has ever investigated this question before the present study.

As the reader will recognize, the findings of my study cannot stand independently in evaluating the functional importance of clinical wisdom. I have asked experienced practitioners about how they live their lives; yet, even if we were to take their answers at face validity, we would not fully be able to say how satisfying these psychotherapists' lives are. To provide a meaningful answer we need a *comparison*. A relevancy design is required that measures the gains obtained from clinical experience and compares it with the wisdom derived from everyday experiences for nontherapists. This relevancy design, of course, requires accurate information about normal adult development. These data, unfortunately, are not easily obtained. While current theories of the human life span are considerably more accurate than classical psychoanalytic theory in describing adult maturation, they nevertheless have a number of significant limitations.

Current information about normal adult development is predominantly impressionistic. Where studies have been done, they have for the most part been investigations of men, not easily extrapolated to the lives of women. Moreover, each of the current theories of adult development, with the exception of Daniel Levinson's (1978), is highly *reductionistic* and culturally bound. All of the theories, other than Levinson's, focus on a single maturational issue that has to be addressed in each adult period of the life cycle. Erik Erikson (1950) gives foremost importance to the conflict between generativity and stagnation as the arena of ego development in the middle innings of life. According to Elliot Jacques (1965) the crucial issue is coming to terms with one's mortality. Martha Wolfenstein (1966) suggests that the transformational task of mid-life is the reworking of one's destructiveness and converting it into mature creativity. Bernice Neugarten (1965) speaks of the development of "interiority"—that is, greater satisfaction and enjoyment in the process of living than in the attainment of specific goals—as the primary required task of maturity.

An apparent major strength of Levinson et al.'s (1978) contribution is that their study followed the vicissitudes of forty men of different socioeconomic classes through each season in the course of their adult life cycle. Yet the empirical basis for Levinson's conclusions about these men's lives must be questioned. The descriptions of what he posits as the four principal tasks of mid-life seem rather similar to the single factor issues of at least three of the theorists mentioned above, and the fourth with the work of Carl Jung. This is to say, Levinson's destruction/creation task is confluent with Wolfenstein's "reworking destructiveness"; his young/old task is easily reconciled with Jacques's "coming to terms with one's mortality"; his attachment/separateness task is similar to Erikson's "generativity versus stagnation"; and finally, his masculine/feminine reconciliation task is precisely the central issue of Jung's theoretical system and the basis for a creative and mature approach to living, which is androgynous, and is reflected also in Neugarten's issue of "interiority." It is not unwarranted to speculate that Levinson might have borrowed the single factor issues of other theorists and posited them in reformulated terms as the basis of his conclusions, because his published study (Levinson et al., 1978) provides little evidence that his view of the principal work of mid-life had been generated on what he actually found in the lives of the men he studied.

In short, the reductionistic theories that are currently available for examining the issues of maturity are inadequate for interpreting the information I received from my respondents. The reports of the senior practitioners interviewed strongly suggest that their issues and concerns are not best explained by a single factor conceptual system or even by a theory that is a string of beads collected from a sundry of research — some clinical and others literary — as have the developmental theories discussed above. What is needed instead is a conceptual system that constitutes the issues of mid-life and beyond as an organic whole, initially derived from empirical research itself, and only then compared and reconciled with the clinical and armchair speculations of other investigators. Lacking such a conceptual schema, it is rather difficult, and perhaps invalid, to examine and discuss possible interactions among and between the polarities conceptualized by Levinson. This is a critical limitation in the explanatory complexity and specificity of his developmental theory.

There are still other important limitations in existing developmental theories of adulthood. Theories such as Erikson's assume that the present capacities to meet developmental tasks are dependent upon earlier maturation that operates in such a logical fashion as to suggest that finally one can happily reach, achieve, and maintain such maturational successes as radiant wisdom and selfless caring and concern for all of humankind. Such a supposition seems characteristic of a selfhood that only a few remarkable people — such as Buddha, Christ, and Moses (at least as religious legends represent them) — have ever attained. In contrast to Erikson's theoretical assumption, the implications of my interviews support Levinson et al.'s (1978) contention that the developmental issues of any one period of adulthood inevitably reemerge in subsequent age periods. The problems of mid-life and the years beyond bear painful witness to this recognition. In the later seasons of life one experiences not only *typical losses* of previously achieved physical and intellectual capacities and development but also frequently an undoing of aspects of one's personality structure due to social and emotional setbacks, such as the loss of a mate or serious financial setbacks.

Admittedly, my strongest criticism of all of the major current theories of adulthood (with the exception of that of Heath (1991)*, which must be examined separately because unlike the others his is

---

*When Heath indicates that the most mature people are characterized by fewer dominant themes in their lives than are less mature people, we begin to recognize the limitations of his study. While it may be true that there are many successful people who steadily pursue a limited number of goals in their lives, this doesn't

not conceptualized in terms of life phases and major developmental tasks) is based on my clinical experience. In my view, human behavior is not impelled from negative or pathological motivation. People act in such a way as to render their experience meaningful for them at that moment in their lives (I will provide the basis for this central tenet of my view on adulthood presently). In contrast, the single factor theories of adulthood (and to some extent Levinson's as well) describe the middle seasons of a person's life in artificially extreme terms that present the important issues of a person's life as "good" versus "bad" options. How else can one regard Erikson's absolute dichotomies of mid-life as "generativity versus stagnation" and senior maturity as "ego integrity versus despair" or that of either succeeding or failing to rework one's destructiveness, as posited by Wolfenstein? These theories reflect the mainstream of psychological theory, which has emphasized psychopathological trends in how people, for the most part white and well-educated males, live their lives rather than taking heed of the constructive and creative mainsprings of all human existence—including that of women and people from cultural backgrounds different from that of the investigators.

A MULTIDIMENSIONAL THEORY OF MATURATION

In the remainder of this chapter I present a multidimensional theory of the maturational issues of adulthood. In order to address the limitations of current theories of adulthood, my theory consists of five existential polarities that exist in dialectic interaction, posited in such a way as to provide a logical sequence and highlight the interrelationship of adult issues.

---

seem to represent truly creative people, who are compelled to seek out ever more complex and innovative ideas and activities.

Indeed, when we more closely review Heath's research sample we find that none of his subjects is described as creative, although several of them are shown to be highly adept at adaptive problem-solving.

Unlike Heath's more mature subjects, the more skillful and creative psychotherapy practitioner, in questioning how he and his patients live their lives, continually risks his present state of certainty in order to discover "deeper" truths about the human condition. Like Erikson, Heath perceives maturity as an all-or-none achievement. Wisdom and maturity are always relative states of being, responsive to the demands of that period of development in which the person finds himself. In each new stage in the life cycle, although life experiences are brought along, new life structures require requestioning and responding anew to unique demands.

The idea that the conflictual struggles of seasoned practitioners might be usefully conceptualized by a multidimensional dialectic process originally came from my interview with Dr. Y. He spoke with acrimony about the vicious political battles in which many of his senior colleagues are engaged, causing considerable conflict in their professional relationships. When I asked about the effect of their destructive power ploys on the way they practice psychotherapy, he stopped and thought for a while; then he said:

I hadn't thought of this before. But perhaps the way these power-driven guys practice clinically has nothing to do with how they conduct the other business in their lives. I say this because I have heard from a number of different people who have been patients of these practitioners that these men are quite compassionate and sensitive analysts in their own offices.

I wouldn't agree that the ways that these men conduct their lives and practices are unrelated, no more than the kind and civilized private demeanors of the Nazi doctors described by Robert Lifton (1986) were unrelated to their inhumanity as concentration camp physicians. But what is relevant in Dr. Y.'s statement is the recognition of the necessity of discarding forever the explanation of complex people, as most psychotherapists undoubtedly are, in terms of their being psychological types. I submit that it is erroneous to assume that any one of us is either essentially power-driven or kind and caring. All of us are many sided. We play not only different roles at different stages of our lives, as Shakespeare indicated, but also at any one time, as Goffman (1959) lucidly argued.

The complexity in our personality makeup results from the *tension of opposites* as we try to come to terms with who we are and how best to articulate our sense of our personal identity to others. In this regard, Jung (1956) is more helpful than Freud in understanding the conflictual issues in the lives of therapists as a dualistic struggle between creative and constructive forces. Indeed, the novel *Tender Is the Night* was a literary exploration by Fitzgerald of Jung's thesis that a person in conflict is strongly attracted to a powerful force in another person that is sensed as a potential counterbalance to one's own overwhelming conflictual desires. The coming together of these magnetically drawn people, Fitzgerald implied, results in the destruction of the apparently stronger but actually weaker personality. I believe that Fitzgerald misread Jung in this regard. Based on the central doctrine of the ancient Greek philosopher Heraclitus, that it is the necessary tension between opposites that is the basis of harmony, Jung (1956) wrote that the striving for wholeness and self-realization requires a dialectic process *within* the personality.

These speculations about the role of a dialectic process in self-realization recall Jones' (1961) attempt to explain Freud's genius. Jones characterized Freud as motivated by an obstinate dualism that pervaded both his thinking and the way that he conducted his personal life. According to Jones, Freud was forever fighting pulls between scientific discipline and philosophical speculation, as well as a number of other contradictory tendencies that included a capacity for both brilliant critical insights and facile gullibility. Jones (1961) explains the dualities in Freud's personality as follows:

> Now Freud had inherently a plastic and mobile mind, once given to the freest speculations and open to new and even highly improbable ideas. But it worked this way only on the condition that his ideas came from himself; to those from the outside he could be very resistant, and they had little power in getting him to change his mind. I was at first puzzled by this resistiveness to outside opinion until I hit on what I consider to be the explanation of it. An intuition, soon confirmed by evidence, told me that side by side with Freud's great independence of mind and skeptical criticism of ideas was also a concealed vein of the very opposite — his resistiveness was a defense against the danger of being too readily influenced by others. . . . this curious strain in Freud's nature, far from being an unfortunate weakness or deficiency, constituted an essential part of his genius. He was willing to believe in the improbable and the unexpected — the only way, as Heraclitus pointed out centuries ago, to discover new truths. It was doubtless a two-edged weapon. It led Freud at times into making serious misjudgments, possibly even ridiculous ones, but it also enabled him dauntlessly to face the unknown. (pp. 379–380)

Following my rereading of Jones's account of Freud, I interviewed Dr. W. who, when asked if his notions about neurosis and human nature have changed during the course of his career, told me:

I do a lot of writing so I am always reformulating my ideas about myself and my work. It is difficult to give you any one direction that characterizes my work. As I finish one paper I am already criticizing that position in another. I used to be tough on myself. I used to say to myself, "I no longer believe that nonsense. How could I have ever thought that way!" I no longer do that to myself. I now know that I am going to change my views about my work and my life and I feel good about that. It is quite exciting to me. I have increasingly come to believe that it is the novelty of the situation rather than a truth buried deep in the unconscious that makes for constructive therapeutic action. If you start to think about things differently you can go on from there and you need not stop growing.

This creative analyst, similar to Jones in describing Freud, is alluding to the intricacies of the *dialectic process* between stability and change that is essential to self-discovery, natural growth, and maturity.

The language of dialectics gives us a vibrant and complex explanatory set of processes, a fertile context from which to understand human behavior. For example, it is more accurate to describe people who have lived deeply as moving from positions of having known deep love as well as intense hatred than to try to determine whether they actually are warm and kind or angry and cruel. I take the position that a person is not really one "true self," hidden intraphysically, there to be discovered only by sophisticated psychological inquiry. Metaphorically, each of us may be described as consisting of many "selves."

This concept is similar but not identical to what Jung has described as an *archetype*. It is instructive to regard these selves, as Jung did with archetypes, as more or less elastically interrelated patterns of behavior existing between two significant life forces. Also, for the most part, in the Jungian sense each of these selves at any one time expresses itself in terms of a *manifestly operative polarity* and a *latent potentially operative polarity*.

From this frame of reference, ambivalence and personal conflict have two major sources. Most often, these are moments in the life cycle when both sides of one of these selves are vying for dominance in order to express their depositional needs. For example, patients in psychological treatment vacillate between intense personal curiosity about their own motivations and a morbid fear of what they might discover and believe that they cannot accept about themselves. Times of greatest crisis are when two or more of these selves are antagonistic to each other. This conflict may threaten the integrity and survival of one's personality, as in the early career of the psychiatrist who disdained desire. His need to feel professionally competent and well-regarded was in violent conflict with his responsibility to respond compassionately to his suffering patients.

In the Eriksonian sense, the side of the polarized self that is most likely to dominate at any particular time is determined by the way that we have negotiated specific identity issues earlier in our lives. However, were this the only operating force in our personalities, behavior would remain largely constant. We cannot understand human growth and creativity unless we recognize that intrinsic to human intentionality is curiosity not only about the external world but also about the polarized selves in our personality. We desire to intimately interact and participate in the lives of each of our polarized selves.

The nature of these interactions are heavily influenced by the developmental issues in our lives at that moment. As common sense should tell us, these developmental issues are best handled by a person who has flexible access to both sides of each polarized self and the resources, such as courage and trust in oneself, to enable these selves to interact constructively and creatively. Moreover, when a dialectic issue is denied or circumvented, serious problems in psychological growth will likely arise.

It also should be pointed out that external crises are not the only causes of tension among the selves. These adverse feelings will ensue even following successful resolution of developmental issues because a growthful personality never remains integrated in the same way for long.

I believe that Freud's (1937) recommendation that practitioners "enter analysis once more at intervals of, say, five years and without any feeling of shame in so doing" was based on his intuitive recognition of the sequence of developmental crises in the lives of psychotherapists. Freud's advice in this matter has been largely ignored, as we found in Chapter 5.

My view of what constitutes these polarized selves differs in some ways from what I understand to be Jung's conceptualization of an archetype. People differ, in Jung's view, as to which specific archetypes are available and operative in their lives. In contrast, everyone shares the existential issues that comprise the polarized selves. Therefore, according to my theoretical position, the question to ask in trying to understand a person is not what is the dominant force(s) in that person's life (which is an inquiry about archetypes), but under what conditions and circumstances does one side of a polarized self dominate rather than another, and what are the potentially constructive and creative energies of the interacting selves that are being fostered at that stage in the person's life. Both resolution of tension and creative expression come from the successful cooperation of well articulated sides of two or more polarized selves.

THE POLARITIES DERIVED FROM BASIC EXISTENTIAL ASSUMPTIONS

I approach the question of what forces in the human condition determine the issues that need to be addressed in mid-life and the years beyond from a small number of existential assumptions. These have been influenced by the theory of personality of George Kelly (1963). Kelly indicates that the dichotomizing of experience is not necessarily a product of the individual's conflictual relation to the world or to oppositional instincts within his psyche. According to Kelly, duality is an essential attribute of thinking itself. An individual creates his own way of perceiving the world by formulating his experience in terms of *constructs* that have varying degrees of predictive efficiency. The cardinal principle that guides the use of one construct rather than another is that *the need to make sense of one's being-in-the-world* organizes all our other needs and motives.

These constructs are, of course, not passive speculative beliefs. They are implicit strategies for taking action so as to live most *meaningfully*. Therefore, those constructs that offer an individual what is to him the best *predictive* options for understanding his experience will be the most attractive. Some of these options will be transient and represent only the convenience of the moment. Others will be more enduring in terms of their roles in presenting options for living one's life meaningfully and well.

My theoretical system implies that the overriding task for the individual at each stage of the life cycle is to make sense of one's existence in terms of one's *personal identity*. An individual's personal identity is a complex enterprise. It consists of not only the sense of whom one currently is but also includes beliefs and desires about who one should be and might become. From this perspective every action and interaction on one's part may be judged in terms of the information it provides for either substantiating or disconfirming the self that one desires to be. Where there is a congruent fit between the experiences of the *tested self* (e.g., the import of one's senses about the circumstances of one's life) with the images, fantasies, and intentions of one's *desired self*, a feeling of competence and well-being accompanies these experiences. A lack of congruence results in shame and discontentment (Goldberg, 1991).

The existential task of monitoring one's personal identity involves basic questions to be answered in dialectic fashion in terms of the five spheres of possibility in human existence. Each of the existential polarities are described in the pages to follow. In reviewing these dialectic issues one should keep in mind not only the specific context of these issues but also their interaction with the other polarized selves.

EMOTION AS GUIDE TO PURPOSE

Traditionally, there has been a need in the behavioral sciences to develop a comprehensive theory of the role emotions play in adult development and to integrate this theory with existing knowledge of cognition, volition, and manifest activity. Until recently, notions in the behavioral sciences about the nature and manifestation of emotion have served us poorly. Personality theory is deficient without a unifying concept, like emotionality, which takes human intent and purpose into account. Recent theories of personality provide a better understanding of the constructive and purposive action of emotion (Goldberg, 1991).

Each of us craves a sense of meaning for our existence. The recurring theme of human existence is the self's striving for personal identity, significance, and unification. In closely examining human experience, we inevitably discover that the evocation of deeply encountered feelings fosters the processes and provides the directions toward which we aspire as purposive beings. Emotions are essential to human purpose. When we are in contact with our emotions, we have an unswaying gauge of what we seek from our existence.

Meaning is derived from our passions. Our passions induce us to become involved in our existence. Why else would we continue to struggle with "the slings and arrows of outrageous misfortunes," other than in the fervent desire to participate in the full enrichment of our passions? (Goldberg, 1980).

The Sensory-Cognitive Self

In a primitive state of development, emotions happen in relation to pleasant or aversive events in which the person finds him or herself.

TABLE 9: Issues of Self-Realization in Adulthood

FIVE EXISTENTIAL SPHERES

1

Developmental Issue:	**SENSORY-COGNITIVE**
Existential Question:	"What kind of person do I believe myself to be?"
Dialectic Process:	**Certainty versus Curiosity**

2

Development Issue:	**COURAGEOUS-CREATIVE**
Existential Question:	"What experiments, exercises, and ways of being will help me become the person I intend to become?"
Dialectic Process:	**Discovery versus Industriousness**

3

Developmental Issue:	**INTUITIVE-EMOTIONAL**
Existential Question:	"What fears and conditions are interfering with my experiencing all aspects of my existence directly?"
Dialectic Process:	**Vulnerability versus Power**

4

Developmental Issue:	**PASSIONATE-SOCIAL**
Existential Question:	"How do I use my relationship with myself and with others to become the person I intend to become?"
Dialectic Process:	**Self-Awareness versus Peer Influence**

5

Developmental Issue:	**VOLITIONAL-SPIRITUAL**
Existential Question:	"If I am the person I intend to be, how do I put my values into action?"
Dialectic Process	**Compassion versus Accountability**

One experiences oneself, as if looking at oneself as an object, as happy or sad or whatever. One's moods are abrupt and often extreme. Typically, however, the person's demeanor is one of indifference or even subtle discomfort.

The developmental task in this stage of seeking self-realization is to address the existential question: "What kind of person do I believe myself to be?" To answer this question meaningfully one must *become aware of possibility*. This process involves examining the assumptions one makes about how one is presenting oneself in the world.

Becoming aware of possibility requires that the self reorient itself toward its own bodily being. As the self becomes appreciative of its assumptions, it discerns how these assumptions induce postures—

physical, psychological, and spiritual. These postures filter the self's experience in the world. To find out who one is one must contact one's innermost needs. To do this the self must transcend its external postures, closing off from its own typically undifferentiated and fused relationships with others and get into itself. To experience its own natural bodily rhythms, unfettered by the need for socially structured expression, the self must turn away from objects-in-the-world for intending. When feeling bodily sensation — whether pleasant, anxious, fearful, or whatever — the self must turn away from seeking objects for fantasized or active engagement. The self can fully contact its self-processes by focusing on its bodily sensations, emptying its consciousness of thoughts and instead centering on internal sensations, allowing its soma to become accessible to its own energies.

Finding who one intends to be involves taking a reconnoitering toward one's experience. This endeavor requires relating one's place in the world to one's internal processes, along the lines suggested above. The sensory-cognitive self utilizes the polarities of **curiosity** and **certainty** in seeking to address its concern about who one believes oneself to be.

Curiosity is an intrinsic propensity with which all but an unfortunate few enter the world. It may be defined as the capacity for inquisitiveness and the accompanying feeling of wonderment about what one does not know. Curiosity involves the willingness to suspend judgment and to explore with passionate interest the conditions of one's world. Certainty, on the other hand, is concerned with what one believes one does know. It is an assuredness of belief; an unwillingness to suspend judgment, ask questions, or subject one's beliefs to doubt.

In seeking possibility in order to address who one believes oneself to be, both curiosity and certainty are appropriate and necessary attitudes. As practitioners of the examined life, we can never be satisfied with our certainties and firm beliefs. We must periodically question everything we cherish and hold firm. At the same time, as practitioners we need a faith that our mission is a worthy one. Our confidence in our work can serve as a sanctuary of safety and trust for our patients until such time as they find their own beliefs. Consequently, to practice fully and well we need to take a stand on important affirmative values. While curiosity furnishes the raw material for fostering a sense of who we are, certainty provides a consistent vision of self, giving our lives direction and purpose. Maturational difficulties can interfere, however, with an adaptive balance between these essential polarities of self-monitoring.

The following brief vignette illustrates how an aging practitioner's unwillingness to examine the issues of the meaning of time in her own life had serious deleterious consequences for her patient.

Nora, the aging analyst introduced in Chapter 2, had been abroad for a number of weeks of professional meetings and vacation. Lois was her analysand of five years and a promising young actress, who had been planning to leave the coastal southern community in which she lived when she completed her analysis in several months. Lois also had planned, with Nora's knowledge, to marry her fiancé, Richard, at that time. During Nora's absence, the teaching position in the north that Richard wanted so badly was offered to him. He would have to relocate shortly. He asked Lois to move with him to the north. To facilitate her move he found for her a drama teaching position at the university. The position was full-time and would begin at the same time as his did. She viewed the move north as a propitious opportunity to get on with her life.

When Nora returned she viewed Lois's behavior quite differently. She regarded Lois's decision as childishly impulsive. A well-analyzed person, she pointed out, should take into account her analyst's possible response, even after she had terminated analysis. Lois had not, Nora pointed out, recognized that Nora, not Richard, knew her best. Since she had depended upon Richard's unwise counsel, rather than hers in this very important decision, she obviously was too dependent on Richard. Consequently, she said their marriage, at least at this time, was unwise.

As an analytic patient, Lois had made a commitment to not make any important decision in her life without discussing it first with her analyst. Nora expected Lois to honor her commitment to not leave town until her analytic work was completed. The work obviously was not finished, Nora sternly told her. With the full gravity of having been an analysand of an analyst who had been analyzed by Sigmund Freud himself, she indicated that she would not permit Lois to act out by prematurely terminating and thereby to destroy five years of arduous analysis.

That evening when Lois entered the apartment she shared with Richard, the impish, infectious smile that typically basked her face was absent. "I can't move yet or get married right now," she said as she slumped into her worn easy chair, which she had planned to give away when she moved.

"You can't let her do that to you! You are an adult. We've spoken about this many times. You and I know that you have outgrown her. And what about our relationship? You said you were ready to close the book on your analysis. Besides, she is an elderly woman—she might terminate with you before you do with her."

Richard was posing a question that had concerned Lois when she first met with Nora in consultation for an analysis. Nora's response at the time (and whenever the issue had resurfaced), was to indicate that she was in perfect health and as able an analyst as ever.

Richard left the coastal community without Lois. Sadly, their relationship had come to an end. Nora was able to facilely fit this information into her firm beliefs about the role of psychoanalysis in human affairs. After Richard left, she told Lois, "Aha! So you see that your analysis endures even when your passionate love affair does not!"

Human purpose is only meaningful to a finite being—someone who will someday cease to be. An individual gains purpose by seriously grappling with his/her finiteness and mortality. Without appreciating the meaningfulness of time in human existence, an individual's attempts at a meaningful definition of self as a finite, purposive being are doomed to futility. The crux of our existential dilemma is that, while the use and structuring of time are essential in seeking meaning in human existence, the fear of contaminating and dissipating precious remaining moments by probing the implications of time has led some aging practitioners, like Nora, to deny and, in so doing, to misuse their own and their patients' precious time. By not recognizing the reality of human finiteness, they separate and insulate therapy from real life.

"A complete analysis" is an unrealistic dream, as most of the psychoanalytic masters (with the notable exception of Ferenczi) recognized (Goldberg, 1975). Practitioners who are afraid to be curious because of what they might find are compelled to take positions of rigid certainty, denying their patients the right to question their practices. Their patients are then discouraged from their most important therapeutic task, which is to gain the legitimacy and necessary skills in the art of self-examination without which discovering one's own intentionality is not possible. Chapter 10 discusses the implications of denying one's limitation of time in the impediments to self-analysis.

The Courageous-Creative Self

Human purpose involves a struggle with ambivalence and pain. The most difficult moments in trying to find oneself are when the individual must push into the murky, veiled, lonely emptiness and stay persistently with the unknown self in trying to find what is hidden inside.

The developmental task in this phase of self-realization is to address the existential question: "What experiments, exercises, and ways of being will help me become the person I intend?" The self responses to this question by *turning toward possibility*, by daring to go beyond experiences to which it has typically confined itself. To feel deeply, as in psychic pain, is to become aware that I hurt because *I care*. The self accentuates its caring by making moment-to-moment decisions to endure and to do something with what it is experiencing — that is, not to ignore, neglect, or suppress what it is feeling. The discovery of caring through staying with one's hurt — and in so doing finding the means for becoming who one intends to be — was moving expressed by the poet, Anne Sexton:

Creative people must not avoid the pain that they get dealt. I say to myself, sometimes repeatedly, "I've got to get the hell out of this hurt." But, no, hurt must be examined like a plague.

In order to find the best ways of expressing itself, the self may use the dialectic polarities of **discovery** and **industriousness**. Discovery involves coming to know about something that previously was not directly experienced. Discovery is a further step in the process of being curious. It exceeds curiosity, in a similar way that being creative is the refinement of experimentation. Industriousness, in contrast, is the skilled or clever exploitation of creative discoveries, usually those found by someone else. Inventors are generally not good merchants and vice versa.

Both the scientist and the artisan are interested in discovery. Each approaches the question of what may be found differently. The scientist asks about the *truth* of an action; the artisan wonders where the action will take him. As psychotherapists, we may be artisans or scientists; rarely, are we both. This is even true of the most outstanding practitioners. Both Freud and Jung had some characteristics of the artisan in them; but each was far more an artistic scientist. Both found fascinating new paths of psychic treasures, leaving the refinement of these discoveries to their more exacting and obsessive followers.

Just as discovery is vital to our profession, being industrious has its place. For example, one could take either side in the argument as to whether it was Freud or Jung who made the greatest contributions to psychology and be able to present convincing evidence. On the other hand, it seems less arguable that Freud attracted far more able collectors and systematizers than did Jung. These industrious practitioners have much to do with Freud's popularity.

In trusting what we learn from our patients, some practitioners are better at reformulating and converting others' ideas into principles of sound practice. Others are better at making new clinical discoveries than following tried and true methods. Still others, among those who have at mid-life become highly successful and famous, have cast off the love of discovery through the years, as one might the letters of an early romance. There is a famous analyst who practices in town. He is reputed to conduct about fifteen therapy groups a week, comprised of about fifteen patients each. Many of his "patients" are therapists themselves. This analyst is famous for his wit and conceptual brilliance. It would appear that, because he has so many patients and he is so enjoys being an entertainer, he hasn't been able to keep track of all those supposedly under his wing. A patient of his for the last twenty years, a senior practitioner in charge of the clinical training of hundreds of therapists, has—for as long as he has been in treatment with the "entertainer"—been involved in serious psychopathology. He lives in the home of a former patient and has been sexually involved with numerous students he supervises. As a director of training, he responds to therapists who are sexually involved with their patients with an unconcerned smile. Several years ago I treated a patient who was a casualty of the clinic this senior practitioner directed.

Industriousness is valuable in the practice of psychotherapy when it promotes sound guidelines that permit practitioners to mature wisely. It is a dangerous polarity to become fixated on, when the practitioner, in turning out a popular product, simultaneously eschews careful investigation of the consequences of his or her work.

The Intuitive-Emotional Self

By this phase the self has some notion of its identity and has liberated its vitality through a courageous willingness to present its identity to others. The self, however, still has not affirmed its investment to possibility. The self has to commit its vitality to focus on a single preferred possibility among others. For this to happen, the self must go beyond its immediate experience of the world as it is presently constituted and formulate a wish or idea of how the self wishes to constitute itself in the world.

The developmental question in this phase is: "What fears are interfering with my experiencing my existence directly?" The self responds
to this question by *making an emotional decision about possibility*.
The need for meaning in one's existence cannot be reduced to a need
for factual knowledge. Factual knowledge has validity only to the
extent that external reality is allowed to define the personal identity
of the self. Fear is a separate source of vitality that cannot be learned
about from the outside. Fear accelerates the heart and drives the
blood through our veins. We may be more alive in our fearful moments than at any other time. The quest for meaning, therefore,
requires sensing what trepidations the self is willing to encounter in
coming to know itself. Consequently, self knowledge requires an
awareness of the choices we make. Decisions are evaluations. As we
express our preferences, so we choose our loves and hates. To know a
person we must appreciate not only what he has experienced, but
more importantly, what he has done to make his life more congruent
with his intentions.

The dialectic between **vulnerability** and **power** suggests that a vita-
lizing strength of character is gained by those who are able to weather
their limitations and vulnerabilities and in so doing openly tolerate
their fears. Stated another way, the capacity to move freely across
dialectic continuums, together with the skill flexibly to blend tendencies from two or more existential spheres, enables practitioners most
successfully to examine their personal identities, putting into action a
way of life that is lived fully and well.

A senior practitioner's worst fear came to pass. A patient in his
analytic group had a friend in the sheriff's office who told him that
his therapist was being blamed for having caused a patient's suicide.
The patient brought this up in the group. Sitting there, the therapist
felt devastated by embarrassment. He no longer regarded himself as a
therapist but as an upset, overwhelmed, and ineffectual person. Tears
came to his eyes. He could neither conceal them nor even wipe them
away. In his despair, he felt too exposed and inadequate to trust the
instinct to hide from condemning eyes.

Asked about his tears, he spoke of having let down his patients and
the people closest to him. The patients in his group might have questioned his professional competence and decided that it was foolish to
remain with him. Instead, to his great surprise, each of them expressed appreciation for what he had done for them and sincere
caring for him. One of the group members, a therapist herself, posed
what she regarded as an important analytic consideration. Each of

the people in the group, she pointed out, had come to him with serious difficulties in their capacity to relate intimately. How is it, she asked, that each is able to demonstrate a genuine capacity to care for him if he has failed them as a therapist? Indeed, another patient added, by not hiding his pain and trusting the group members' responsiveness to his vulnerability, he was showing confidence in them and furthering the important work of developing compassion that he had fostered in the many months (in some cases, years) of therapeutic endeavor.

The Passionate-Social Self

The self requires dialogues with other selves in order to reveal its own intentionality to itself. A thing in itself can only be itself. Creating new possibilities requires engagement with other selves in order to actualize the potentialities in each.

The developmental task in this phase is to address the existential question: "How do I use my relationships with myself and with others to become the person I intend to become?" In responding to this question the self utilizes possibility by *valuing immediate engagement*. Since the dialectic process in this phase involves a balance between **self-awareness** and **peer influence**, the engagement may be with self or with another. This dialogue involves a *letting go* to permit what the self is experiencing at the moment to emerge—in terms of its values, wants, and vulnerabilities. This letting go requires a caring for oneself without the defensive-protective stance of constraining other selves. Letting go is the preferred stance of the passionate self in being open to experiencing its avoidances rather than seeking reassurances and certainty about its assumptions. The self receives caring from another by sharing its preferences and concerns, freeing the other to relate to the self as the other experiences the self. "Reality" exists for the self only by virtue of the way it relates with other selves. Communication, therefore, is an extremely powerful vehicle. When the self directly and courageously addresses interpretations by other people that are constricting or inauthentic definitions of what the self intends for itself, the self is enabled to constitute itself in a constructive way. This often is most easily stated than achieved.

Both sides of the passionate-social self are problematic. We live in a world of few external certainties. Often we feel compelled to look into ourselves for the meaning of our experiences. At the same time, our uncertainty in our own feelings and judgments forces us to look to others for direction. In this regard, clinical experience, be it with a severely disturbed patient or even a disturbed person we encounter in our everyday world, can troublingly test the dialectic between our passionate and social self.

Psychotherapists want to be perceived not only as competent practitioners but also as caring and compassionate human beings. Few of us involved in the practice of psychotherapy view ourselves as lacking caring or compassion. Some years ago a medical school that was considering appointing me as full professor received a letter from an obviously highly disturbed woman who accused me of a possessing sinister power to visit people through time and space. This woman, whom I shall call "Rita Stone," was an attractive school teacher I had met at a cocktail party. Sensing at the time I met her that she was emotionally disturbed, I excused myself and walked away several minutes later. I was surprised, therefore, to receive from her two phone calls a couple of weeks later. The first was direct and innocuous. She told me that she had enjoyed meeting me. She also told me that she was changing her job and was going for an important interview. I didn't expect to hear from her again. But, unfortunately, I did! The second call was briefer and very strange. She told me that she was going to get a job with sincere people and would never have anything to do with people like me again. I had no idea where she was coming from or what she was talking about.

Because of her letter, I was asked by the medical school to provide a written account of my contact with Rita Stone. I was angry and resentful that this bizarre event was happening to me. It was unfair, I felt. Like most of my colleagues, I go to considerable trouble — often beyond any reasonable professional responsibility — to be of assistance to disturbed people like Rita Stone in their darkest hours. I had tried to be empathic and concerned when I spoke with her — and she was not even my patient. Now my appointment at the medical school as full professor was being jeopardized.

Unfortunately, because I didn't understand the dynamics of shame as I do today, I didn't seek out some consultation with a trusted colleague to discuss the matter. I felt that, if I were really a competent practitioner, I would be able to work this problem out by myself. I didn't do too well initially. The self-recriminations for allowing this situation to happen continued to hound me.

Finally, I realized that a large part of the problem for me came from the overidealized position of being a therapist, especially a senior practitioner. As psychotherapists, who are held up by the public as supposedly those who are par excellence in handling human affairs, we are ready targets for resentment, attack, and ridicule from disturbed people, especially if these, as I suspect of Rita Stone, have had some unfortunate experience with mental health professionals in the past. I surmise that she tried to rid herself of her shameful helplessness from her past painful experiences by expressing her anger at me.

This clinical understanding might have assuaged my feelings of *vulnerability*, if I experienced the *compassionate* polarity of the *volitional-spiritual sphere* (discussed later in the chapter) and felt sorry for her because she was so clearly disturbed. On the other hand, someone else might have responded to this existential dilemma with an indignant sense of not allowing her *irresponsible* and destructive behavior (the second polarity of the *volitional-spiritual sphere*) to remain unpunished; that person might have consulted an attorney about possible litigation. On the other hand, my response after the initial shock and feelings of resentment was a *cognitive* one. I was highly *curious* about how I had become unwittingly involved in Rita Stone's psychopathology.

Social critics, such as Susan Sontag (1964), believe that it is both inaccurate and unfair for clinicians to maintain that people bring about and even "encourage," at some subliminal level of intent, their own misfortunes. I, too, would have preferred to see my having been treated unfairly as the result of a paranoid person arbitrarily selecting me as her target. But my clinical sense would not allow me so easily to get off the hook. I was compelled by some inner psychological integrity to set aside my anger and resentment and seriously explore whether in some implicit way I had encouraged her bizarre accusation.

After many years of conducting therapy groups and working with volatile couples, I was aware of the *intersubjectivity* of human interactions and how people mutually mistreat one another. After considerable rumination, I realized that I probably had conveyed a number of mixed messages to this disturbed woman. I had to admit to myself that when we had first spoken at the party I had found her very attractive. From her behavior at this initial contact, these sentiments were evidently reciprocated. Moreover, initially I had found it not in keeping with how I wished to perceive myself to coldly hang up the phone on a highly upset person with whom I was acquainted. I tried to offer some support. Nevertheless, even without fully recognizing her considerable psychopathology, some intuitive part of me prevented me from pursuing subsequent encounters with her. Nonetheless, responding ambivalently, I did not make my intentions sufficiently clear to her. In the intersubjective context, shows of caring and compassion are easily misunderstood by emotionally hungry people.

If this had happened with a patient within a therapeutic situation, it might have had some useful ramifications in helping both the patient and myself differentiate and learn to clearly define the kinds of caring the therapist is willing and able to provide. In the real world with a disturbed person with whom one doesn't have a contractual or personally committed relationship, the intersubjective confusion about what specifically the people involved are willing to provide is highly provocative, difficult to manage, and as this story demonstrates, often outrightly dangerous.

My experience with Rita Stone has had some positive residuals. I am part of the "real" world as well as the consulting room. I must use what I learn from one world to enrich the other. In my subsequent clinical work and my supervision of other therapists, I have become highly sensitized to the importance of precisely specifying how the practitioner is prepared and available to care for the patient during the latter's difficult moments. When such boundaries are missing, misunderstandings, detrimental to both patient and therapist, can result from a male therapist, for example, telling his female patient something to the effect that "I care for you and what you are going through. And I want you to know that I am here for you." Under this provocative shroud, it is easy to slip into an exchange of the therapist's promise to care in return for the patient's inappropriate responses, such as adulation, sexual advances, unquestioning acceptance of the therapist's opinions, and so forth.

Appropriate and meaningful therapeutic power comes from recognizing the limitations of one's ability and willingness to care, and on this basis not promising overtly — or implicitly — to do what one feels compelled to do because of abstract ideals about what is therapeutically compassionate and proper. By understanding one's own intentions and communicating them in a clear way to patients, the practitioner can avoid the intersubjective shaming that took place in the Rita Stone incident.

The Volitional-Spiritual Self

"Freedom," says May (1977), "is most clearly shown in the human capacity to ask questions. Every question implies that there is more than one answer, otherwise it would not be asked."

The developmental task in this phase is to address the existential question: "If I am the person I intend to be, how do I put my values into action?" The self becomes its own possibility by articulating and acting on the experiential possibility that if, when I act, I assume that the course of action I take is authentic to my being the person I intend to be, then I will experience the freedom to choose among possibilities.

The polarities in this phase are **compassion** and **accountability** (alluded to earlier). Each of these polarities has a significant place in our system of morality and values. Outside of specific situational contexts, however, rarely can we determine the preferable course of action between these values. This can be illustrated in the following hypothetical example: Dr. A. is a criminologist. He believes that the world would be a better place if each of us upheld with courage and fortitude the highest standards of personal responsibility. On the other hand, Dr. B., a clergyman, feels that the social problems that plague us would be best resolved if the ways we treated ourselves and others were informed by liberal amounts of tolerance and compassion.

Ethical and moral issues involved in being a practitioner were a major concern of several of those who answered the questionnaire. The following vignette touches upon the dialectic between compassion and accountability.

"Sid Fallon," an experienced analyst, psychotherapy educator, and writer, was telephoned by a young psychiatrist, Arnold Miller, for a consultation. During the initial interview, Miller matter-of-factly told Fallon that he was embroiled in a scandal at the hospital at which he worked. He had been accused by a couple of the female patients he was treating in the outpatient clinic of taking sexual liberties with them. The director of the hospital investigated the accusations, regarded him as guilty without even a formal hearing of the hospital ethics committee, and promptly dismissed him. To make Miller's life even more difficult, the hospital director had encouraged the women to take legal actions against Miller. The psychiatrist calmly indicated to Fallon that the accusations were entirely false. They were due not only to tranferential distortion, he told Fallon, but also to a misunderstanding by both of these women about Miller's therapeutic techniques.

Sid Fallon did not hesitate in agreeing to help. He had always taken pride in his ability to work constructively with even the most difficult cases. When he pressed Miller during their second consultation for precise details about what actually had happened to cause the patients to levy charges of unethical behavior, the psychiatrist admitted that it was true that he had come on sexually to the women. In the context of treating Miller on a three-times-a-week basis, Sid went to considerable trouble for Miller. He spoke in private to both the attorney retained by the women and to the State's Attorney — men he knew well from his work as a respected forensic psychologist. He worked out an agreement where money was paid out of court to the plaintives but no criminal charges were made against Arnold Miller.

Inevitably, the psychotherapist's office is a place of shame. The patient who comes to us is ashamed because his presence in our consulting room is experienced as an indication of his incompetence as a person. Moreover, our very presence magnifies his shame. Our being there during the recitation of his secrets compels him to reflect painfully upon unworthy and mortifying aspects of himself (Goldberg, 1991).

When a person has been repeatedly shamed about his capacity to be competent, acceptable, and cared for, as Arnold Miller had been, he will be caught up in a conflictual dialectic, vacillating between the desire to be just "ordinary," with the common flaws and limitations of every human and an accentuated desire to be "extraordinary," beyond needing to prove his worthiness and value as a person over and over again. A person like Arnold Miller poses considerable danger to those with whom he is involved. He will seek help from those who can insulate him from the need to be special. But at the same time, someone's tolerance of his shameful actions and the disturbing fantasies that fuel his behavior may painfully remind him of how different and inferior he is to that person. Consequently, a therapist's kindness paradoxically is experienced by people like Miller as an especially cruel form of hatred. It confronts the patient with an accentuated sense of being different and inferior.

He may try to protect himself from his self-hatred, from being reminded of his limitations, by not allowing the ostensibly caring and concerned practitioner to reach him in a meaningful way. He also tends to project his hatred toward someone who has character traits he desires and has failed to develop by his contemptuous behavior. He has the "ear" and, astoundingly often, credibility with colleagues. In this venue he will circulate lies and misinformation about his therapist. Miller did this by reproaching Fallon to other practitioners and turning Sid's most sincere and valiant efforts to help him into therapeutic blunders and insincerity.

During dinner parties, professional meetings, and departmental conferences at the university, Fallon became aware of his colleagues' side-glances in his direction, accompanied by muffled snickering. He did not know what to make of his colleagues' changed behavior in his presence. It was only when a colleague alluded to an aspect of his private life that the speaker should not have known that Sid suspected that Miller may have discussed distorted information from what Fallon had self-disclosed in an analytic session.

He questioned Miller the next time he saw him. The patient nonchalantly admitted what he had done. He seemed unremorseful; moreover, he coldly told Fallon that as an experienced practitioner Sid should not get so easily upset.

It was not so much what had been done to him, but who had done it, that most upset Fallon. He had worked arduously for Miller and had been caringly available to him. And for this Miller had violated and betrayed him. He had stolen from him his integrity and a faith that by being personally and professionally responsive to his patients he would be rewarded with respect and appreciation by patients and colleagues alike. His faith in the tenets of his profession had been derisively returned as foolish naivete.

When Sid angrily insisted that his patient examine the sources of his sadism, Miller stormed out of the office, never to return. The lies and misinformation circulated by Miller continued.

Practitioners are largely unprotected in dealing with attacks against their reputation by their former patients. Whereas we are free to publicly confront and pursue litigation against a colleague who slanders and misrepresents us in his capacity as a colleague, we don't have that same right with colleagues if we become their therapists. It would appear that we have to abrogate at least some of our legal rights and protections in our roles as therapists. This is because it would be difficult, if not impossible, to defend ourselves against a patient's slander and still maintain our pledge of confidentiality about what we know about the patient and what actually transpired in the therapeutic hours, unless a patient initiated charges of misconduct against the practitioner.

THE INTERACTION OF THE POLARIZED SELVES

For each of us in mid-life and the years beyond, the particular dialectical issue with which we are confronted has to do with existential questions that we are at that moment wrestling with in terms of our personal identity. In complex conflicts these polarities rarely operate in isolation from one another. For example, a practitioner can use his *responsibility* to his patient unwisely in the *intuitive-emotional* sphere by not respecting the patient's *vulnerability* and overriding it with the *power* of his knowledge and expertise. It also is possible that this practitioner does not trust *self-awareness* (neither his patient's nor his own) and is forcing his influence on the patient to reinforce his own need for *certainty* about what he believes. As practitioners of the examined life, we all have experienced achieving our greatest self-discoveries when we felt most lost and became openly *curious* about where we were. We also know that therapy, if rendered without *compassion*, can be devastating to the patient. I still vividly remember, when I was a candidate in a post-graduate psychotherapy institute over twenty years ago, sitting behind a one-way glass and watching a seasoned practitioner conducting psychotherapy with a very fragile, suicidal young woman. The patient became inordinately upset during one of the sessions. She was in tears, screaming that the therapist was like everyone else in her life who claimed to want to help her but was actually indifferent to her real needs. She jumped up, promising never to return to therapy because her life wasn't worth holding onto. My classmates and I, concerned about the upset woman, called out for the therapist to go after her. I don't know if he heard us. I don't think that it would have mattered to him. He sat there and didn't move. In our post-session with him he justified his actions on the basis of his theoretical position. His theory said that if he went after the woman he would be manipulated time and again. The patient never returned.

But then neither must we denigrate *certainty* as an important factor in curative therapy. Some of our greatest achievements as a civilization have been from people who firmly hold onto an idea when it is not safe or popular to do so. Our firm trust in therapeutic beliefs can be for many disoriented patients a safe sanctuary of steady and reliable support in which to find and forge their own convictions— provided that our certainty about our own ideas includes the encouragement of the patient's own *self-awareness*.

There is no single true and correct response to the developmental issues of mid-life. The conceptualization of a dialectical process between two different psychological tendencies that are neither positive or negative in themselves is a response to my conviction that all behavior emanates from a health striving—the intention of making sense of one's being in the world.

In the next chapter I explore the issues involved in the seasoned practitioner's renewal.

— nine —

THE WISDOM OF
SELF-RENEWAL

Grow old along with me!
The best is yet to be,
The last of life, for which the first was made,
Our times are in his hand,
Who saith, "A whole was planned,
Youth shows but half; trust God: see all, nor be afraid!"
. . .
Therefore I summon age
To grant youth's heritage
Life's struggle having so far reached its term:
Thence shall I pass, approved
. . .
So, take and use thy work;
Amend what flaws may lurk,
What strains o' the stuff, what warping past the aim!
My times be in thy hand!
Perfect the cup as planned!
. . .

—Robert Browning

Once I stood on a very high summit. Below me everything appeared quite small but nevertheless perspicuously set out. I felt content in having found an unique perspective on the world. As I turned to leave I happened to glance behind me. I was startled to realize that out of earlier sight stood a much higher hill. Undoubtedly, if I were to climb the hill in back of me I would find an even broader view. I felt a sense of nausea in having been deluded by my short-sightedness. This analogy cogently speaks to the life and practice of the seasoned practitioner.

The growing maturity of seasoned practitioners modifies their youthful values and perspectives on neurosis and human conflict.

Wheelis (1956) has pointed out that the young practitioner tends to believe that psychoanalysis and psychotherapy are finely attuned rational tools that can enable him or her to successfully come to terms with all types of human suffering. Wise, mature practitioners, as I have tried to demonstrate in this book, have a less fervent faith in their own psychological insight and expertise. They place more trust in their patients' inner wisdom and the healing capacity of compassion, decency, and common sense than they did as beginners. They also recognize more creative ways of adapting to aging than they imagined as youths.

THE NEED FOR SELF-RENEWAL

Along with the satisfactions of practicing psychotherapy come stresses and frustrations. At mid-life, practitioners may experience these stresses more acutely than at any other time in their careers. It is at mid-life that many practitioners realize the full implications of their career choice. Many report that their depressive feelings have their source in early family dynamics that have compelled them to take a caretaker or healer role (Mccarley, 1975). In mid-life they come to recognize their residual resentment at having been cast in this capacity long ago in their lives. It also is at this time that they feel depleted from the losses of mind, body, spirit, and relationship that darken the mid-life season for everyone.

The important task of mid-life is a paradoxical assignment. In the face of the loss of the safe and familiar, the qualities of life and one's own person that have for so long been taken for granted, the practitioner must recognize and hopefully respond to opportunities for new beginnings. A person at mid-life usually has the time, resources, and experience for renewal of maturity. It is expected that senior practitioners, having for many years practiced the examined life, will scrupulously review what they have accomplished in their careers and on that basis determine what there is still to learn and to achieve in their clinical practice.

In this chapter I will comment on some of the time-honored ways practitioners have undertaken this review. But before I do this I must speak first to the reader who believes that this chapter is simply beside the point, insisting that personal psychotherapy is the only real answer to the practitioner's professional and personal concerns. I would respond by reminding the reader of what we have already learned in this book about the developmental issues of maturity. We have seen that there are professional issues that may be helped by personal psychotherapy but for which therapy alone is not sufficient. Also, there are professional and personal concerns with which the senior practitioner may be struggling which the respondents' statements on their questionnaires suggest are not best handled by psychotherapeutic treatment. Just as many of us tell our patients that there is real life outside the consulting room, such that some issues should not be relegated to personal therapy, so, too, for us as practitioners the answers to life's vicissitudes cannot be fully met by the therapeutic session (Goldberg, 1990b).

D. W. Winnicott (1960), the British analyst to whom one typically can turn for good common sense and reassurance, has wisely pointed out that personal analysis does not free the practitioner from neurosis; rather, it serves to increase the stability of the practitioner's character and the maturity of personality. This, Winnicott (1960) reminds us, is the basis of our professional conduct, allowing us to maintain an effective working relationship with our patients. Nevertheless, professional codes are actually descriptions of an idealized version of ordinary people. Consequently, the practitioner is under continuous stress in maintaining a professional attitude at all times, under all conditions, and at different stages of development as a practitioner and as a person. Consequently, practitioners like Drs. A., Q., U., and Z. who report to be the same person when they are practitioners as they are in their private lives, probably experience less strain in their clinical work than Drs. O. and P. who feel the need to separate their personal and professional lives, as does Dr. R. as well.

According to Winnicott (1960), even repeated returns to "the couch" do not remove the strain of maintaining an idealized professional role. It is for this reason that seasoned practitioners struggling with the issues and concerns of mid-life and the years beyond need advice, consultation, and support in examining how they are living their lives beyond the assistance offered by personal therapy.

An additional factor needs to be considered. Several of the respondents who struggled with the idea of returning to the couch indicated that too often a highly trained practitioner's pride prevents him or her from asking for the help required. We have been oriented as practitioners—through our training, if not our characters—to handle life's most excruciating problems and suffering in private. It is hardly surprising, then, that a majority of practitioners (both women and men) reported that their clinical practice had either an ambivalent or detrimental influence on their significant relationships. This is not a surprising finding. As I indicated previously, Henry and his associates (1971, 1973) found that most of the psychotherapists they studied felt closer to their patients than to colleagues and family.

Emergencies are almost always the times when we require others' help. Common sense dictates that we need not to be alone in dealing with difficult human issues. As we try to persuade our clients of this simple human reality, so we must persuade ourselves! Collegial interaction is a very important source of support, regardless of whether or not one returns to personal therapy. We can share the most agonizing moments of our practice with trusted colleagues, as many of the analysts interviewed indicated, whether this be in a private consultation, in a peer group, or in collaborative clinical endeavors. Professionally and personally we require collaboration with and support from our colleagues. There are numerous clinical and personal concerns that we do not have to and should not deal with alone. This is true whether the concern is one of self-doubt, an error of omission, or even one of commission, such as a rageful or sexual indiscretion toward a client. Of course, we can handle many of these matters by returning to the couch. The usefulness of the couch, however, often is not immediate. In the meantime, we can turn to colleagues for assistance.

To Return or Not to Return to the Couch as a Moral Issue

As we have seen in the reports of a number of seasoned practitioners, some therapists develop a sense of fraudulence about the examined life. They feel that their commitment to analytic understanding of themselves has not harvested the savory fruits of the well-lived existence that their faith in psychoanalysis and psychotherapy had promised. As young practitioners they believed that their skills as able psychotherapists who could understand the world in a way that ordinary people could not was their investment in the future. Their talent, like fine wine, had to age before it could be properly savored. However, over the years their examination of their work has taken unexpected paths. They have come to recognize that psychological inquiry does not hold an exclusive franchise in separating illusions from existential truths. Their despair comes from the realization that as knowledgeable as they are about human relations, their commitment to the examined life has not led them to living a more vibrant life than those people who appear to be less self-examined.

One of the most difficult questions confronting the disillusioned practitioner who regards his theory and practice as fraudulent is whether to try to resolve his troubles by returning to the couch or by some other means. There is a thorny problem involved in this question: can a practitioner successfully find answers to questions about the limitations of his practice by using that practice to evaluate his dissatisfactions? For in doing so is not the practitioner tacitly confirming that all his questions and doubts are not real but countertransferential? Wheelis (1962) cautions us about the folly of assuming that despair is synonymous with pathology. For if this were true, then all moral problems would be dismissed and all troubling issues relegated to psychological problems. For the disillusioned practitioner attendance in a peer consultation group with trusted colleagues seems the most prudent.

PEER SUPERVISION GROUPS

As practitioners move into private practice from agencies and large institutions, where colleagues are readily available for social and professional exchange, they often feel the increased isolation and existential exhaustion that was so frequently mentioned by the seasoned practitioners I questioned about the major perils of mature practice. Private practitioners may be deprived of opportunities to openly examine their own and their colleagues' personal values and existential concerns. The practitioner needs the opportunity to represent him/herself in all aspects of self rather than being confined to circumscribed attributes; yet, the demands of private practice typically limit the therapist's roles.

When one lacks opportunities for exchange with trusted colleagues and for the evocation of deeply encountered feelings about one's work and aspirations, the strains of continuous clinical practice frequently develop into feelings of being "burned out," evoking disillusionment about one's work, its importance, and its impact. Under these circumstances, values seem vacuous pursuits bereft of satisfaction, and personal and professional endeavors lacking in direction and purpose.

Many senior practitioners in the throes of this existential malaise seriously consider leaving the practice of psychotherapy. Some actually do. Peer supervision groups, if purpose and process are well-attended, offer one of the best opportunities I know for personal and professional growth and revitalization for the seasoned practitioner.

In a previous book (Goldberg, 1990b), I have discussed at length the numerous important issues that must be efficaciously addressed to best insure a viable peer supervision group experience.

Co-therapy as Personal Growth

For me working with other experienced and creative practitioners in various clinical endeavors has proved an excellent way to renew enthusiasm for clinical work. Practitioners will be best able to use collaborative therapeutic endeavors if they are prepared in a visceral way to achieve parity and share their deep fears and fantasies with their co-therapists during their work together. I have discussed a model for the collaborative clinical endeavor elsewhere (Goldberg, 1990b). Another model for collaborative personal growth for experienced practitioners was offered a number of decades ago by Warkentin, Johnson, and Whitaker (1951).

In addition to an organized peer group and structured collaborative efforts, there are still other means of support for the practitioner that I have discussed elsewhere (Goldberg, 1990b, 1991) and it would be repetitious to repeat here. However, the issue of challenging cases deserves some discussion.

Challenging Clinical Cases

No matter how successful, every practitioner needs to take on a few different types of patients (especially difficult ones) to keep growing. The statements of several respondents who were seriously disillusioned with their clinical work earlier in their careers and were able to overcome their despair and find revitalization by changing their perspectives on neurosis and human nature suggest that it is useful to experiment with different therapeutic approaches. Like travelers who learn about their own culture through the eyes of foreigners, practitioners can learn much about their own practice in this way, in addition to being invigorated by occasional journeys into previously unknown psychic terrain.

In short, in mature practice one needs to have a variety of patients and clinical activities. This prevents the practitioner from "assembly lining" his or her professional life. The contrasts between different kinds of patients creates a variety of perspectives on the human condition. As we have seen with Alan, the psychiatrist who disdained desire, a perspective on human existence becomes artless and even dangerous whenever the practitioner assumes a position of having finally and with certainty figured out neurosis and human nature. Contrasts among patients can constructively challenge firm beliefs (Goldberg, 1990b).

Ironically, in another sense the seasoned practitioner needs to be highly selective in choosing patients. The practitioner has the personal responsibility—to say nothing of personal right—to pursue personal growth in such a way as to remain finely attuned to his patients. Unlike the beginner who can profit from clinical work with just about any patient, experienced practitioners need to ask themselves whether working with certain patients is in their best self-growth interests. Many of the practitioners responded to the question about the limitations of therapeutic dialogue by indicating that much of their own boredom, stultification, and even despair stems from having allowed themselves to bear, over extended periods of time, responsibility for and commitment to men and women who dwell only in their own shadows and whom they intuitively believe will always be, despite the best therapeutic efforts, too fearful or damaged to live fully for themselves, let alone share a vital presence with anyone else.

Dr. Q. began her practice before she had children of her own. Earlier in her career she enjoyed working with young children. Now that she has children at home she doesn't want to work with other people's children at the office. One of the most important lessons she learned as a mature practitioner, she told me, was that there are some patients with whom she is not at her best; she doesn't want to work with them and feels no need to defend her preferences.

The Psychotherapist Has No Season

Many seasoned practitioners hold onto the saddle with the same rein to the very end. It would appear as if there were nothing they wanted to do or that they believed that they could do well enough to pursue as an avocation or second career. It is prudent to consider that for some practitioners being a psychotherapist is one developmental stage in their lives and they need to move on.

Early in my career I had a friend, a man close to sixty. He was an eminent practitioner, the former president of a psychoanalytic society. He had spoken in the past of being ready to retire. He had complained that the winters in the Midwestern city in which he practiced were getting more unbearable each year. He wished to retire to the Middle East and pursue his great interest in history and archeology. But he was unwilling to do so even when he was financially able. For my friend, as well as for many others, to pursue another field would be tantamount to admitting to themselves and to others that they had failed in their careers as analysts. In order to protect their career integrity, they look upon being a psychotherapy practitioner as a final stage of their lives. Sadly, shortly before he was to leave for an archeological dig in Israel, my friend suffered a fatal heart attack.

How long should practitioners stay in their careers? It is difficult to say. Unlike most other professions, the career of psychotherapist has no season. Athletes, whether they wish to accept the inevitable or not, are aware nonetheless that their season is short. They can only thrive in a young person's time. If their pride doesn't tell them, then their physical capacities and performances surely will. Even in the academic professions and performing arts there is a natural progression from doer, to teacher and mentor, to theorist and chronicler, to administrator, to consultant as emeritus. In contrast, psychotherapists, similar to the other profession of spiritually oriented service providers, the clergy, can and often do stay on the firing line until the very end. Since the profession is generally more shaped by altruistic and moral issues than financial interests, the sense of personal identity is more tied into one's career than with most other professions. To give up one's career as psychotherapist, even to substantially transform it, may require serious modifications in how one regards oneself and what one is willing and able to do with nonpractice time.

ten

CONCLUSION:
TRIUMPH OVER ADVERSITY

If it had not been for these things
I might have lived out my life
talking at street corners to scorning men.
. . . .
Now we are not a failure.
This is our career and our triumph. Never
in our full lives could we hope to do such work
for tolerance, for justice, for man's understanding of
    man
. . .

— Bartolomeo Vanzetti, "Last Speech to the Court"

The sixty-four individuals who speak out in the study reported in this book enable us to enter — what is notoriously difficult for the observer — the consulting rooms and the private lives of seasoned practitioners of psychotherapy. Their self-reports suggest that most seasoned practitioners, especially master practitioners, feel pleased by their career choice. These practitioners appear to be caring, sensitive, and dedicated to their patients' welfare and their own personal growth and professional proficiency. At the same time, it is alarming that there are a considerable number of experienced practitioners for whom "the light has failed." These are practitioners who have had unsatisfactory personal analyses or psychotherapy, find self-examination unproductive or even frightening, feel isolated from friends, family, and a sense of community, and even sense that they have been betrayed by the psychological theories and world views they were provided with as beginners. They regard the underpinnings of their psychotherapeutic practice, psychoanalysis, as providing them with an extremely pessimistic account of human affairs, thereby, not enabling them to understand and deal with their patients in a compassionate and meaningful way. These practitioners find that psychoanalysis, even more than other therapies, lacks a theory of action — that is to say, a methodological system for making constructive processes happen in therapeutic sessions. They also feel poorly prepared by their training to compete as professional entrepreneurs. The most frightening finding of all is that there may be some senior practitioners who, even though prospering financially and professionally, trivialize their disenchantment about clinical work by regarding it as an interesting pastime, but not one that will significantly improve the quality of their patients' lives.

How do we answer the central questions that have guided the investigation: Are mature psychotherapists, despite their extraordinary preparation for examining the human psyche, like other people of their own age? Or do they, as a result of a personal character that has drawn them to their work and/or the nature of the work itself, respond differently to their developmental issues than do others of their age?

I believe that the complexity of the therapist's task is such that the competent mature practitioner has to be simultaneously like other people his or her age and quite different. Robert Lindner (1954) indicated that:

Neither the science of psychoanalysis nor the art of its practice depends upon extraordinary agencies. As a matter of fact, the only medium employed by the analyst is the commonest instrument of all — his own human self, utilized to the fullest in an effort to understand its fellows. (p. xiii)

What I take Lindner to have meant is that, in order to be empathic and fully available, practitioners need to be able to readily identify with the hopes, fears, ambitions, and travails of their patients. This open identification enables them to learn from their patients. As a younger practitioner I learned from patients older than I about experiences I had not yet encountered. For example, I heard a variety of different perspectives on marriage from my patients before I experienced my own marriage. Even seasoned practitioners can continue to mature by being open to experiences of their patients that they will never have themselves. To some extent all of the female patients I have worked with have provided access to issues I will never directly experience.

This suggests that there is an essential substratum of enlightened mutuality in the self-realized practitioner. This mutuality is based upon the recognition that genuine friendship has through the millennia been the sine qua non of psychological healing. Genuine friendship cannot be one-sided (Goldberg, 1991). Reciprocity is integral to the enrichment of human experience. Each of us in dyadic interrelationship — therapist and patient, teacher and student — needs to feel that he or she has given something valuable in return for what has been received (Goldberg, 1990b).

Stanley Greben (1984) provides a moving account of the mature practitioner recognizing the importance of mutuality in the developmental rites of passage in terminating an analysis. In describing his visits with Olive Cushing Smith in Baltimore after he terminated analysis with her, Greben wrote:

> In the subsequent fifteen years, until her death, I visited her in her home another five or six times. She was always pleased to see me, and continued to follow with great interest the course of my career and my life. In turn I welcomed the increasing opportunity to give to her the friendship and interest and occasional companionship which were now, because of her advanced age and increasing physical limitations, so important to her.
>
> When I had been the one who was more in need, and hence more to receive than to give, she had given to me, comfortably and easily. When it was time for me to move on, she accepted that with comfort and grace. When eventually our positions were reversed by the passage of time, neither of us had difficulty in adapting to the change. (p. 117)

On the other hand, to not only deal authentically with patients but also offer them resources in reframing conflict, the seasoned practitioner must have a somewhat different perspective from them and experience more existential options than they do. Master practitioners teach *reframing* strategies in which the meaning of a situation is changed by modifying the context of the event, even if the factual situation remains the same. Reframing involves skillfully blending different modes of thought. When there is too much emphasis on doing, one's sense of who one can become, rather than who one "is" is lost. When there is too much concern with one's inner world, effecting a withdrawal from the world, one remains only a potential emergent being. Hidden in this stance is the shameful risk of living as less than perfect. As a "potential" one need never actually test who one wishes to be. In this regard, then, the enabling practitioner asks his or her patient to courageously examine his/her life. Courage, in this sense, is to know one's limitations, to accept one's self as less than perfect, to live to the best of one's ability and to come caringly together with others to heal the wounds of loneliness and the dread of human existence. The master practitioner deepens the patient's creative dialogue within self and with others, so that this person is vibrantly involved in his or her existence when alone or with another.

The experienced practitioners in the study tell us that they developed an enabling world view not from the dubious wisdom of their theory but from having faced important existential issues countless times with different patients. This enables some practitioners, presumably the eminent senior practitioners foremost, to mature earlier than other people.

The point of view I delineate above suggests that the troubled practitioner is likely to be one who rarely experiences or examines him/herself differently from those who come to consult with him or her. Or, even more unfortunately, he/she may be a practitioner who believes him/herself to be vastly superior to his or her patients and, as such, is out of touch with the abiding issues of patients. Enlightened mutuality obviously is impossible in this imbalanced therapeutic arena.

Are the practitioners I interviewed wise people? I sensed that each in his or her own way was highly astute. For most, this wisdom was low-key, based upon the conviction that each person must find his or her own answers, because no one has *the answer* for anyone else. Their agreement on this issue appeared to center on the recognition that whatever the particular answer might be for anyone, it needed to be struggled with within the context of the oppositional forces within and from outside of the self. Most importantly, these eminent practitioners seem to be telling us that it is wise for us to regard the need to reconcile oppositional forces in one's lifespace as an unique opportunity for authentic development and enriching human experience, rather than as an unfortunate obligation of life. This is a notion that I have emphasized in my theory of dialectic self development (discussed in Chapter 8).

Even the most sensitive and astute senior practitioners can get locked into despair if they don't appreciate the propitious opportunity dialectic development offers us. Take the statement of Allen Wheelis (1956). He tells us that the problem of intimacy is for many analysts the principal determinant to their careers. But rather than regarding being a psychotherapist as a superb way of coming meaningfully to terms with this need, he regards it as a narcissistic defense. The problem, he indicates, is "the conflict between the tendencies that lead to closeness and the fear that is evoked by closeness." Becoming a psychoanalyst, he maintains, is a compromise between these vacillating needs. The problem with this type of conceptualization of human emotion (as discussed in Chapter 8) is that it casts emotions in negative connotations and regards the ostensible desirable need — a longing for closeness — as a reaction formation defense against an unexamined conflict — the fear of being overwhelmed by the closeness of the other. The need for solitude and self-examination is as legitimate a need as is the need for closeness, depending of course on the place one is at in one's dialectic development. The sense of boredom and stagnation, which if unaddressed results in despair, comes from seeking similar satisfactions and accomplishments across different stages of development.

As I have discussed elsewhere (Goldberg, 1991), those who "specialize" in their lifespace — giving inordinate attention to matters at which they excel, while at the same time avoiding activities that they don't do well — are shame-vulnerable people. They have much to tell us about why it is so painful and difficult to explore our own inner world alone or with another. My clinical and personal experience as I will try to demonstrate suggests that the fear of self-discovery has to do with the taste of what *is yet to be* — being alone on our own death journey.

When I began thinking about writing this book, I also started my own self-analysis. To assist me, I began a daily journal in which I examined my thoughts and feelings in my writing the book; especially what unexplored issues might be motivating me. The first entry in my journal stated:

> I am starting this journal today. I hope to use it both as a means of examining my own personal and professional issues and as material for the book I am writing about the seasoned practitioner. It is hard to consciously admit that I need to write a book on the mature practitioner. It is, in a real important sense, saying "good-bye" to youth. And yet, as a psychotherapy practitioner for twenty-five years, I realize that not to admit to the need to examine the issues and concerns of mid-life leaves me an unwitting prisoner of their influence.

Writing in my journal did not proceed as I had initially hoped it would. While my patients have found it quite useful through the years to keep daily journals to capture fleeting thoughts and feelings, I myself found it difficult to keep up a daily commitment to my self-chosen task. This was a commitment that required me to take the time to sit quietly for at least a half-hour a day and ponder my inchoate inner promptings and to describe them in detail. I found it tempting to invent excuses to attend to other matters. Nevertheless, for most days for about three months I managed to keep a log.

Then a seemingly trivial clinical interaction with a patient I treated for about a year, after she had attended a psychology course I taught, startled me.

One of the most disconcerting moments for me as an experienced practitioner is realizing that I am still acting out conflictual motives that I had believed that I had already worked through earlier in my career. The patient told me in a session that she had attended reluctantly that I viewed her "as a money machine." She had called me three and a half hours before her therapy session to say that she was feeling ill and didn't think that she should have a session that day. Because she just had taken a three-week break from therapy, I had suggested that she should come in for her session. She pointed out that I should have indicated that she was responsible for her session and left it up to her. She was a business person, she said. She could accept the responsibility of paying for her sessions. Money had been a conflictual issue for me when I began my practice. But, perhaps, I had not (the phase that my free associations presented me with) "yet crossed the line."

In closely examining my feelings about the incident, I discerned among my reactions an emotion that my clinical work with hard-to-reach patients revealed to be *shame*. I experienced myself as flawed and incompetent in some important way. I also remembered that I had felt this way about a year previously when I was thinking about whom to dedicate my book on shame (Goldberg, 1991). I thought over those people in my personal and professional life who had been helpful and supportive to me in my career. I remembered with special fondness a supervisor from my clinical internship whose personal kindness and caring presence with patients and interns alike has been an inspirational model for me long past that of more theoretically astute supervisors whose knowledgeable words I have long forgotten. I had told myself in earlier years when I thought about my apprenticeship as a practitioner that one of those days I would look up this special supervisor's address and write him. What I kept denying in my procrastination was that my mentors were not immortal. What is not said or done today may be left forever lost. When finally I did look up the former supervisor's address, I sadly found that he had died some time before.

I thought at first that the severity of my reaction to the patient who had confronted me was due in part to that experience being a shame displacement associated in some way to not having acknowledged the kindness and wisdom of friends and teachers in the past. However, if this were the dominant substratum of my feelings of shame as a practitioner, then there would follow a facile flow of entries in my journal of other moments in my life and my career in which I felt ashamed for not having acknowledged past kindnesses. To the contrary, I was shackled in my self-examination. My free associations were replete with the words and the deeds of my patients and people in my personal life who had struggled with whether to end their lives.

The relevance of these associations to feeling ashamed as a practitioner made no immediate sense to me. But some other associations did. They arose when I visited Dr. V.'s house to interview him for this book. Sitting in his office waiting room I remembered with mixed emotions my childhood experiences with psychoanalytically trained European teachers.

It was in a boarding school, with its German accent and the conveyance of the love of books, Mozart, and the outdoors that I first heard the mention of psychoanalysis. Also, there I first experienced the capacity of the psychoanalytic mind-set to reach the inner recesses of the psyche. My teachers, who had fled to the United States from the Nazi holocaust, were well-educated and trained in Gestalt psychology and psychoanalysis. They conveyed an understanding of human behavior that was for me mysteriously powerful. They seemed able to put into articulate words the intrapsychic messages that sustained periods of silence for my classmates and me.

My experience with these European teachers is closely related to my reason for pursuing the research investigation described in this book. As a child, I felt that these psychoanalytically sophisticated people, at times, did not use their knowledge wisely. However, these teachers were not trained to be psychotherapists. Interviewing some of those reputed to be the most capable of the psychoanalytic profession allowed me to find out whether having the intellectual and detective talents to be able skillfully to descend into the dark realm of the psyche could also be influential in developing mature wisdom.

My experiences with these European teachers are related to my reasons for becoming a psychotherapist. At some subliminal level, psychological knowledge presented to me a means of both understanding and escaping the confusing conflicts of my nuclear family. Studying psychology lead me to a career in which I could be independent of my family. Because psychology had such a salubrious effect on me I was as a beginning therapist uncomfortable about being paid. My most gratifying clinical year was my internship in which I assumed that the clinical skills I was developing would enable me to experience the world in a way that ordinary people could not. The fact that I was paid a minimal wage, so low that I was actually eligible for welfare payments, was no problem for me because my sacrifice was my investment in the future.

In remembering how I experienced myself in my twenties as a beginner in my career as having an unforeclosed future, as contrasted to my present perspective of mid-life with a more limited future, I recognized that the passing of my supervisor in his mid-life testified to an important part of the mystery of the impediments to self-discovery. Earlier, I had reexamined the literary classics in writing about the role of shame in the history of ideas (Goldberg, 1991). What I remembered most vividly was Leo Tolstoy's powerful dramatization, in *The Death of Ivan Ilych*, of death as the ultimate shame because it provides undeniable evidence of our powerlessness and defeat as human beings in being able to control our ultimate fate. Shame, as an ontological emotion, therefore, issues from the profound despair of having no future moment as an existent being.

Nietzsche (1887) explained the efforts of those who seek superiority through eminent wisdom as the wish to be aligned with God. As an Übermensch, there is a magical belief that one can defeat death. However, to be aware of what one does not know is to experience one's finitude and mortality. Self-knowledge, therefore, is the estranged sibling of magic. As such, self-discovery imposes a threat to the wish to be able to transcend the limitations of human finitude. The unconscious, as Freud (1900) stressed, is *timeless*. Because of the sense of no limitation of time in the unconscious, there is no negation of possibility in those recesses of the psyche that are still unexplored. Magically, not to know is not to be limited. We rationalize our procrastinations in self-discovery by assuming that we will live forever and therefore have unlimited time. In the light of day, the awareness of human limitations derived from self-knowledge soberly confronts our magical strivings for immortality through omniscience. There-

fore, shame, in its ontological role, if not understood as a constructive guide in alerting us to what crucial issues we are denying in our
lives, prevents self-discovery. And as such, I believe, it is a major
impediment to self-analysis.*

Giving up magical beliefs, difficult as it may be, affords us the
benefits that surrendering all other illusions provide. Gould (1978),
as I mentioned earlier, believes that the major false assumption of
mid-life is that "There is no evil or death in the world." When we free
ourselves from this assumption's deceptive security, we find that the
vulnerability it exposes in us has life-affirming potential. He points
out that liberation from the fallacies of youth

> gives us access to the deepest strata of our minds that we have
> ever examined. It's our final natural opportunity to deal with the
> deeply buried sense of our "demonic badness" or "worthless-
> ness" that has curtailed us from living as legitimate, authentic
> creatures with a full set of rights and a fully independent adult
> consciousness. (p. 218)

There are few efforts in life that produce as acute a sense of shame
as the recognition that one is incompetent in striving for caring and
intimacy. Wheelis (1956), referring to psychoanalysts as not only
permitting but demanding isolation, casts a needless shaming rendi-
tion of a desire for solitude which may require a reconciliation with
the desire for intimacy but is not good or bad in itself. Our career
choices I strongly believe are unwitting efforts to make possible such
developmental reconciliations.

Developmental reconciliation is related to the theme of those interviewed overcoming adversity in their lives. There was strong evidence
that all of the senior practitioners interviewed, with the exception of
Dr. R. and possibly Dr. P., became psychotherapists because earlier
in their lives they felt rather dissatisfied with the directions their lives
were following. Some viewed themselves as footloose in their early
lives. Others regarded their lives in a tragic light. It is not surprising
that most felt that, although they were not following any conscious

---

*If self-analysis is actually an indispensable but poorly understood professional and
personal guide of the practitioner, then more attention needs to be given to it in the
practitioner's training. Its utilization should become a prominent component of the
practitioner's personal therapy, as well as integral in his/her supervision and training.

dream in becoming psychotherapists, no other career could have been as congruent with both their reparative and proactive growth needs. In trying to come to terms with themselves, these master practitioners have found ways of helping others understand themselves. They appear able to create highly responsive emotional dialogues in which unexpected and novel psychological processes are experienced. For these practitioners, therapeutics and learning are interrelated. In this way many of those interviewed have returned, with a vastly greater understanding, to an early career interest. Teaching is of considerable satisfaction to all who I interviewed. Several started out to be teachers but became enchanted by psychoanalysis along the way to the classroom.

For most of the practitioners interviewed the career choice of psychotherapist also has a strong spiritual side. They appear to believe that popularity, material wealth, social and political power are empty substitutes for the existential doctrine that knowing oneself and others compassionately and intimately is required in order to live fully and well. They have come to believe that sharing one's psychological insights in a compassionate and courageous way is a sign of tempered wisdom. They hold that there are emotional ingredients to wisdom that technological knowledge does not have. Wisdom has a "generosity of spirit" that philosophers through the ages have underscored. Such wisdom consists of compassion, decency, and common sense, qualities that few of us are fortunate enough to appreciate early in life. In the course of being a practitioner over time we are daily confronted with the lives of our patients, many of which are painfully devoid of these qualities. The course of aging as a practitioner increases the chances of more fully appreciating that which is essential to living fully and well. In short, although being an experienced psychotherapist doesn't guarantee us wisdom, it does give us an excellent opportunity for it.

Opportunities for wisdom, however, are rarely afforded us in a passive stance. Wisdom often requires a paradoxical attitude of catalytic receptivity. *Courage* (mentioned earlier in this chapter) is one of the most important of these catalytic stances, for without courage the unexplored regions of the psyche will not be explored. Courage provides the practitioner with the passion to become a *tested self*. One guides another only by being native to similar terrain. Only the tested, especially those scarred and flawed, can inspire the fearful. Those who have been sheltered from the need to express their desires or have

cowered in the underbrush of their own personal journeys have neither a compass for the brave nor a sturdy walking staff to bolster the
unsteady gait of the fearful.

In keeping with the Eastern notion of wisdom (discussed in Chapter 6), master practitioners can be differentiated from other experienced therapists not so much by the possession of a fount of expertise
as by the willingness to live more fully in the light of their own self-
discoveries. For them the past may not be over, it may not even be
past. Their vibrance comes from the maelstrom of continual self-
discovery. Scientific knowledge, on the other hand, never gives us
immediate insight into ourselves. At best, it tenders a vicarious ap-
proximation of our inner lives as viewed from the role of the unrisk-
ing observer.

If the practitioner has not lived fully, what can he or she offer
those who seek a guide but an inane and illusory expertise? One does
not respond wisely to the dilemmas and opportunities in another's
life by simply possessing factual knowledge about how the other
became fearful and why some of our yearnings may be unsatisfied.
The wise practitioner guides the seeker by the maturity of his or her
tested self — and in so doing teaching the seeker how to blend the hard
realities of life with passionate and romantic dreams.

An examination of the human condition suggests that our awareness of human possibility is as much invigorated by romantic passion
as it is foreclosed by desperate terror. There is actually no acceptable
reason for continuing to live except that we want to exist. The meaning we crave for our existence is derived from our passions. Our
passions induce us to get involved in our existence.

Thus, human existence is doubled-edged. While revealing the tragic substratum of life, human consciousness, at the same time, provides us with a romantic imagination and fantasy to transcend the
given state of affairs of our present world. Our romantic nature is our
most redeeming attribute. It enables us to love and care for others
and to strive for what we believe.

For master practitioners, the romantic imagination is afforded by
the experiences of their tested selves, which provide practitioners with
the larger vision. There are in every person's life, said the novelist
James Hilton in *Lost Horizon*, moments when we glimpse the eter-
nal. The wise practitioner draws on those moments to create a vision
of hope from the phoenix of adversity. The master practitioners I
interviewed have fashioned, piece by piece, and tested by personal
application an overriding philosophy of life that is both more practi-

cal and more creative than the world views that guided them as youth. They are practical in being straight-forward and optimistic, articulating their convictions in everyday terms that are less involved with the "real" reasons and motives for behavior than with what they and their patients are willing to do about their intentions and dissatisfactions. They are creative in selecting as their existential models for living deeply what seem to be the best insights from other people's lives (including their patients'). They appear to perceive reality not as a single entity but as a series of existential options that invite the question that Nietzsche (1887) recommended we use to examine all philosophies of life: can it be lived fully and well?

I must admit that the answers some of those interviewed gave to their existential concerns sounded quite simplistic to me. But what was undeniable is that their psychological convictions enable them to touch others' lives in caring and beneficial ways they had not regarded as important or were not capable of fostering as younger practitioners.

APPENDIX

The letter and questionnaire to follow were sent out to 200 experienced psychotherapists.

The list of issues found on p. 155 comprises the concerns that I pursued in the interviews with the twelve prominent analysts. Each interview was rather different from the others. Which issues were more routinely broached, which were emphasized and pursued in considerable detail, and what additional questions I brought up that I had not originally planned, were a product of the unique chemistry that constitutes open-ended interviews.

DR. CARL GOLDBERG, F.A.P.A., F.A.G.P.A.
LOBBY "C"
305 EAST 24TH STREET
NEW YORK, NY 10010

I am writing to you because you have been identified as a practitioner who is an eminent and articulate senior psychotherapist.

Psychotherapy articles and books have not been written for the seasoned practitioner. Yet, there are serious issues (and even perils) that each mature psychotherapist, inevitably, must face. These may be issues that the mature practitioner had not anticipated when he or she entered the profession. As you know, this is because many of the dilemmas of practice are quite difficult to communicate in words. Some can only be found by personally experiencing them.

Since so little empirical data exist (not even much impressionistic material) on the important concerns to the mature practitioner, I am writing seasoned psychotherapists for their assistance in furnishing this information.

The information that I will gather will be reported in a book that I am writing for W.W. Norton & Company. I wish to emphasize in this regard, I plan to use most of the data anonymously. Any material I plan to identify as to its source I will first write for permission to the practitioner who furnished it. If I don't receive permission I won't identify the source.

If you would like information about my findings I will send them to you prior to publication.

Thank you in advance for your assistance!

Sincerely,

Carl Goldberg, Ph.D.

Enclosure: 1. Questionnaire
2. Stamped addressed envelope

Questionnaire on Being a Seasoned Practitioner

In order to render this questionnaire more meaningful to me please answer the following:

Your name

Your educational degree: Master's _____

Doctorate _____ M.D. _____

If other please describe

The "school" of psychotherapy with which you most closely identify (include more than one if applicable).

Please describe your postgraduate training:

The number of years you have been a psychotherapist _____

The number of years of full-time practice _____

Where you received your training as a psychotherapist:

Hospital _____ Clinic _____ Counseling center _____

If other please describe

1. As a seasoned practitioner, please list what have been the significant issues, concerns and dilemmas that you have encountered in practice that you did not anticipate before entering the career of psychotherapist (perhaps not even as a beginner):

2. Is psychotherapy an impossible career insofar as there are inherent limitations to therapeutic dialogue? If so, what are these limitations?

3. What do you believe to be the perils to the practitioner and the iatrogenic effects of psychotherapy to the patient?

4. Have you ever struggled with whether to return to the "couch"? If so, what enabled you to resolve this issue?

5. What has been your experience with self-analysis?

6. Have your views on neurosis and human nature changed during your career? If so, how?

7. What have been the most important lessons you have learned from your patients?

8. What effect has being a psychotherapist had on your relationship with family, friends and a sense of community?

9. Have there been satisfactions in your practice that you had not anticipated as a beginner? If so, what are they?

10. Do you have a "personal myth" that has directed the way you practice and how you live your life? If so, what is it? If it has changed during your career, how has it done so?

11. Please define what the term "Master Therapist" means to you:

12. Please list those books and articles that you found the most helpful in shaping your work as a psychotherapist:

THE INTERVIEW

1. Education

2. School of psychotherapy

3. Postgraduate training

4. Years as a psychotherapist

5. Years of full-time practice

6. Where interviewee received training as a psychotherapist

7. Interviewee's childhood and adolescent dream

8. Was the dream of youth fulfilled?

9. What are the factors influencing their fulfillment?

10. Has the interviewee's way of practice changed over the years?

11. Expectations interviewee had entering the field

12. Were these expectations met?

13. Significant issues as a mature practitioner not anticipated when interviewee entered the profession

14. Developmental factors in interviewee's life — affecting practice

15. Have views on neurosis and human nature changed over the years?

16. What are the perils of practice to psychotherapists?

17. What are the iatrogenic effects to the patient?

18. Is psychotherapy an impossible profession?

19. What are the limitations of therapeutic dialogue?

20. What is the disillusionment of practice about?

21. Is disillusionment something everyone goes through at mid-life? Or does it have some particular relevance to being a psychotherapist?

22. Has the interviewee ever considered another career?

23. Considered another career after practice?

24. Mentors important in the interviewee's career

25. Has the interviewee ever struggled with going "back to the couch"?

26. If so, what resolved the issue?

27. Experience with self-analysis

28. Personal myth that has directed the interviewee's life

29. Has the personal myth changed over time? If so, how did it change?

30. Most important lessons learned from patients

31. Effects of being a practitioner on family, friends, and sense of community

32. Satisfaction not anticipated as a beginner

33. What are the mid-life issues and tasks of the practitioner?

34. Why has so little been written about mature practice?

35. What is a mature practice?

36. What is a master practitioner?

37. Is there anything else I should be asking?

38. Which other articulate and wise seasoned practitioners should I interview?

ANNOTATED BIBLIOGRAPHY

Following are concise summaries of thirty-six important books and articles relating to the issues of being a mature practitioner. Some of these references are written specifically about the psychotherapist and others concern the issues of mid-life and aging in general.

Bermak, G. E. (1977). Do psychiatrists have special emotional problems? *American Journal of Psychoanalysis, 37*, 141–146.

Bermak, a San Francisco psychiatrist, surveyed 75 psychiatrists in the Bay area. The conclusions of the survey were that psychiatrists do have special emotional issues that are specific to them and their work.

Burton, A. (1970). The adoration of the patient and its disillusionment. *American Journal of Psychoanalysis, 29*, 194–204.

Burton examines factors in the disillusionment process that precede the therapeutic maturation of the practitioner. He contends that these factors are attempts by the practitioner to come to terms with unfinished aspects of self.

Burton, A. (Editor) (1972). *Twelve therapists: How they live and actualize themselves*. San Francisco: Jossey-Bass.

Twelve literate, provocative, and revealing autobiographical accounts of eminent psychotherapists enable the reader to follow the significant developmental issues in the lives of these practitioners as they become master practitioners.

Burton, A. (1975). Therapist satisfaction. *American Journal of Psychoanalysis, 35*, 115–122.

"There is almost a silent conspiracy in the refusal to look at the treatment needs of the psychotherapist," contends Burton. He examines each of these needs and maintains that if they are not met treatment will be sabotaged.

Eissler, K. (1977). On the possible effects of aging on the practice of psychoanalysis. *Psychoanalytic Quarterly, 46*, 182–183.

Eissler traces the three major patterns that the analyst's narcissism may take in the aging process. One of these trends results in rigidity, a second in grandiosity and a third increases the desire for knowledge and reduces therapeutic ambition.

Erikson, E. H. (1980). *Identity and the life cycle*. New York: W. W. Norton.

Erikson discusses healthy personality and the problems of ego identity in adulthood from a developmental perspective.

Farber, B. A., & L. J. Heifetz (1981). The satisfactions and stresses of psychotherapeutic work: A factor analysis. *Professional Psychology, 12*, 621–630.

One of the few comprehensive, empirical studies of the working conditions and experiences of psychotherapists.

Farber, B. A., & L. J. Heifetz (1982). The process and dimensions of burn out in psychotherapists. *Professional Psychology, 13*, 293–301.

A second analysis of their 1981 study. They conclude their analysis of their data with the statement: "The primary source of stress for therapists is lack of therapeutic success . . . (and) the nonreciprocated attentiveness and giving that are inherent within the therapeutic relationship."

Freud, S. (1937). In J. Strachey (ed. and trans.) Analysis terminable and interminable. 316–357. *The Standard Edition of the complete psychological works of Sigmund Freud.* Vol. 23, pp. 209–253, New York: Norton.

One of Freud's most famous and, arguably, enduring papers. He indicates that the analyst's self-examination of his own neurosis and the resistances toward his work is a ceaseless endeavor.

Freudenberger, H. J., & Robbins, A. (1979). The hazards of being a psychoanalyst. *Psychoanalytic Review, 66,* 275–296.

A comprehensive review of the types of people who become analysts and how their character structure, training and world view contribute to the disillusionment process.

Freudenberger, H. J., & Kurtz, T. (1990). Risks and rewards of independent practice. In E. Margenau (ed.), *The encyclopedic handbook of private practice* (pp. 461–472). New York: Gardner Press.

A comprehensive and balanced examination of the satisfactions and the limitations of being in independent practice.

Goldberg, C. (1990). Typical mistakes of the seasoned therapist. In E. Margenau (ed.), *The encyclopedic handbook of private practice* (pp. 785–798). New York: Gardner Press.

The thesis of this chapter is that one of the major causes of experienced practitioners' difficulties is that they tend to deny in themselves the very issues they are concerned with in their patients.

Goldberg, C. (1990a). The role of existential shame in the healing endeavor. *Psychotherapy, 27,* 591–599.

A clinical case study that examines the constructive role that an experienced practitioner's feelings of disillusionment had in working with a difficult patient.

Gould, R. L. (1978). *Transformations.* New York: Simon and Schuster.

An impressionistic and literate purview of the adult life cycle. This work is highlighted by the pungent assumptions Gould posits as impeding psychological growth at each of the stages of adult development.

Greben, S. (1975). Some difficulties and satisfactions inherent in the practice of psychoanalysis. *International Journal of Psychoanalysis, 56,* 427–434.

A comprehensive and balanced account of the concerns and the satisfactions of practicing psychoanalysis and psychotherapy. Greben maintains that psychotherapy is "the most human of all activities."

Greenson, R. R. (1966). That "impossible" profession. *Journal of the American Psychoanalytic Association, 14*, 9–27.
  A now classic paper, which emphatically examines the traits, motivations, and skills required of the competent analyst. Greenson also discusses the conditions in the analyst's personal life supportive of functioning professionally fully and well.

Groesbeck, C. J., & Taylor, B. (1977). The psychiatrist as wounded physician. *American Journal of Psychoanalysis, 37*, 131–139.
  According to the authors, the myth of healing indicates that the patient in psychotherapy has healer in himself and the therapist, a patient. The practitioner should be prepared to have his own psychic wounds reactivated in therapeutic encounter if their coming together is to be meaningful and healing.

Heath, D. H. (1991). *Fulfilling lives: Paths to maturity and success.* San Francisco: Jossey-Bass.
  Heath's book discusses a study, in which he followed the lives of a number of his own students since the 1950s in order to ascertain the precise personality attributes and motivations that best insure an adult life of maturity and success.

Henry, W. E., Sims, J. H., & Spray, S. L. (1971). *The fifth profession: Becoming a psychotherapist.* San Francisco: Jossey-Bass.
  The first of two volumes based on the most comprehensive nationwide study of psychotherapists to be conducted. On the basis of data from over 4,000 practitioners, the authors present detailed information about the personal lives and professional practices of psychotherapists.

Henry, W. E., Sims, J. H., & Spray, S. L. (1973). *Public and private lives of psychotherapists.* San Francisco: Jossey-Bass.
  This second volume of Henry and his associates' research examines the backgrounds, training, and belief systems of psychotherapists.

Jung, C. (1989). *Memories, dreams and reflections* (Recorded and edited by Anielle Jaffe). New York: Vintage Books.
  This book is Jung's autobiographical account.

Kelly, E. L., Goldberg, L. R., Fiske, D. W., & Kilowski, J. M. (1978). Twenty-five years later, *American Psychologist, 33*, 746–755.

This report examines the professional careers of clinical psychologists over a period of twenty-five years.

Levinson, D. J., Darrow, C. N., Klein, E. B., Levinson, M. H., & McKee, B. (1978). *The seasons of a man's life*. New York: Ballantine.

This book is a report on a study that followed the lives of forty men from different socioeconomic backgrounds through adulthood. This work is probably the single most important study of men's lives.

Malcolm, J. (1981). *Psychoanalysis: The impossible profession*. New York: Knopf.

In this book Malcolm interweaves the history and basic psychoanalytic theory into her interview of a New York Psychoanalytic Institute trained analyst who gullibly allows Malcolm to interview him in a subtly derisive way.

Marmor, J. D. (1968). The crisis of middle age. *Psychiatric Forum, 29*, 17–21.

Marmor's paper was one of the first and still one of the best overviews of the problems of mid-life. He cogently relates the identity crisis of mid-life to an inability or unwillingness to realistically accept and constructively redirect youthful aspirations to mature projects.

Marmor, J. (1953). The feeling of superiority: An occupational hazard in the practice of psychotherapy. *American Journal of Psychiatry, 110*, 370–376.

According to Marmor, there is no single source of motivation or personality type drawn toward practicing psychotherapy. There are, however, inherent factors that, if not carefully attended, Marmor cautions, adversely effect psychotherapeutic practice.

Marston, A. R. (1984). What makes therapists run? A model for analysis of motivational styles. *Psychotherapy, 21*, 456–459.

Based on the empirical studies of Farber and Heifetz (1981, 1982), Marston posits eight basic motives for doing psychotherapy.

McCarley, T. (1975). The psychotherapist's search for self-renewal. *American Journal of Psychiatry, 132*, 221–224.

McCarley maintains that the depression many practitioners experience at midlife is due to early family dynamics that have become exacerbated by the normal stresses over decades of practice. He recommends several types of renewal that differ from what would be suggested to a younger practitioner.

Rogers, C. R. (1975). In retrospect: Forty-six years. In R. Evans, *Carl Rogers: The man and his ideas*. New York: E. P. Dutton.

In reviewing the course of his career, Rogers seemed to be more dissatisfied than gratified by his colleagues' reception. He offers a perspective in which to view his work.

Spensley, J., & Blackner, K. H. (1976). Feelings of the psychotherapist. *American Journal of Orthopsychiatry, 46*, 542–545.

This paper persuasively indicates those inherent stresses in the practice of psychotherapy that are not based on the practitioner's countertransference or neurosis.

Spiegel, J. (1986). Self-concept and the inner life of aging. *Integrative Psychiatry, 4*, 191–198.

One of the few reports by a senior practitioner of how the aging process effects both the professional and personal aspects of one's life.

Valliant, G. E. (1977), *Adaptation to life*. Boston: Little, Brown.

In following men's lives through their adulthood, Valliant examines those mature defenses that enabled men best to successfully love and work. This study is still on-going.

Weiner, M. F. (1990). Older psychiatrists and their psychotherapy practice. *American Journal of Psychotherapy, 44*, 44–49.

Weiner interviewed fifteen older psychiatrists and found that for the most part they thoroughly enjoyed their work. It would be largely for reasons of health and disability that they anticipated that they would stop their work.

Wheelis, A. (1956). The vocational hazards of psychoanalysis. *International Journal of Psychoanalysis, 37*, 171–184.

Wheelis, in a poetic and profound essay, describes psychoanalysis as a profession understood only by those who practice it and then only after many years of experience. He indicates that the actual reasons for entering the field may be incidental to what is central to analytic work.

Wheelis, A. (1960). *The seeker*. New York: New American Library.

This book is a novel about a disillusioned senior analyst who tries to escape his despair through a series of cynical professional projects and vagrant sexuality.

Winnicott, D. W. (1960). Countertransference. *British Journal of Medical Psychology, 33*, 17–21.

Winnicott, in this now classic paper, maintains that our professional demeanor actually is an idealized version of the ordinary person. Personal analysis, he argues, frees practitioners from excessive neurosis but cannot remove human vulnerability. Indeed, Winnicott believes that the practitioner's vulnerabilities are essential to therapeutic sensitivity.

REFERENCES

Bagarozzi, D. A., & Anderson, S. A. (1989). *Personal, marital and family myths*. New York: Norton.

Bardwick, J. (1980). The seasons of a woman's life. In D. McGuigan (Ed.), *Woman's lives: New theory, research and policy*. Ann Arbor: University of Michigan Center for Continuing Education for Women.

Belenky, M. F., Clinchy, B. M., Goldberger, N. R., & Tarule, J. M. (1986). *Women's ways of knowing*. New York: Basic Books.

Bermak, G. E. (1977). Do psychiatrists have special emotional problems? *American Journal of Psychoanalysis, 37*, 141–146.

Burton, A. (1970). The adoration of the patient and its disillusionment. *American Journal of Psychoanalysis, 29*, 194–204.

Burton, A. (Ed.) (1972). *Twelve therapists*. San Francisco: Jossey-Bass.

Burton, A. (1975). Therapist satisfaction. *American Journal of Psychoanalysis, 35*, 115–122.

Chessick, R. P. (1977). *Great ideas in psychotherapy*. New York: Jason Aronson.

Chessick, R. P. (1990). Self-Analysis: A fool for a patient. *Psychoanalytic Review, 77*, 311–340.

Clayton, V. P., & Birren, J. E. (1980). The development of wisdom across the life span. In P. E. Baltes & O. G. Brim (eds.), *Life span development and behavior*. Vol. 3 (pp. 103–138). New York: Academic Press.

Dewald, P. A. (1981). Professional profile. When the analyst is seriously ill. Roche Report. *Frontiers of Psychiatry, 11*, 12–13.

Ehrenwald, J. (1976). *The history of psychotherapy*. New York: Jason Aronson.

Eissler, K. (1977). On the possible effects of aging on the practice of psychoanalysis. *Psychoanalytic Quarterly, 46*, 182–183.

English, O. S. (1972). How I found my way to psychiatry. In A. Burton (Ed.), *Twelve therapists* (pp. 78–101). San Francisco: Jossey-Bass.

Erikson, E. (1950). *Childhood and society*. New York: Norton.

Erikson, E. (1968). *Identity: youth and crisis*. New York: Norton.

Erikson, E. (1980). *Identity and the life cycle*. New York: Norton.

Erikson, E. (1987). *The life cycle completed*. New York: Norton.

Farber, B. A., & Heifetz, L. J. (1981). The satisfactions and stresses of psychotherapeutic work: A factor analytic study. *Professional Psychology, 12*, 621–630.

Farber, B. A., & Heifetz, L. J. (1982). The process and dimensions of burnout in psychotherapists. *Professional Psychology, 13*, 293–301.

Fiedler, F. (1950). The concept of an ideal therapeutic relationship. *Journal of Consulting Psychology, 14*, 239–245.

Fiedler, F. (1951). Factor analysis of psychoanalytic, nondirective and Adlerian therapeutic relationships. *Journal of Consulting Psychology, 15*, 32–38.

Fitzgerald, F. S. (1934). *Tender is the night*. New York: Scribner's.

Fleming, J. (1971). Freud's concept of self-analysis. In I. Marcus (ed.), *Currents in psychoanalysis*. New York: International Universities Press.

Freud, S. (1900). The interpretation of dreams. In J. Strachey (ed. and trans.). *The standard edition of the complete works of Sigmund Freud*, vols. 4 and 5, New York: Norton.

Freud, S. (1912). Recommendations for physicians on the psychoanalytic method of treatment. In J. Strachey (ed. and trans.). *S. E.*, vol. 12, New York: Norton.

Freud, S. (1914). Further recommendations in the technique of psychoanalysis: On the beginning treatment. In J. Strachey (ed. and trans.). *S. E.*, vol. 13, New York: Norton.

Freud, S. (1935). An autobiographical study. In J. Strachey (ed. and trans.). *S. E.*, vol. 20 (pp. 3–74). New York: Norton.

Freud, S. (1937). Analysis terminable and interminable. In J. Strachey (ed. and trans.). *S. E.*, vol. 23 (pp. 209–253). New York: Norton.

Freudenberger, H. J., & Robbins, A. (1979). The hazards of being a psychoanalyst. *Psychoanalytic Review, 66*, 275–296.

Freudenberger, H. J., & Kurtz, T. (1990). Risks and rewards of independent practice. In E. A. Margenau (ed.), *The encyclopedic handbook of private practice*. New York: Gardner.

Gallos, J. V. (1989). Exploring women's development: Implications for career theory, practice and research. In M. B. Arthur, D. T. Hall, & B. S. Lawrence (eds.) (pp. 110–132). *Handbook of career theory*. New York: Cambridge University Press.

Gilligan, C. (1979). Women's place in man's life cycle. *Harvard Educational Review, 49*, 431–446.

Gilligan, C. (1982). *In a different voice*. Cambridge: Harvard University Press.

Glover, E. (1937). The theory of the therapeutic results of psychoanalysis. *International Journal of Psychoanalysis, 16*, 125–189.

Goffman, E. (1959). *The presentation of self in everyday life*. New York: Doubleday.

Goldberg, C. (1973). *The human circle*. Chicago: Nelson-Hall.

Goldberg, C. (1975). Termination — A meaningful pseudodilemma in psychotherapy. *Psychotherapy, 12*, 341–343.

Goldberg, C. (1976). Existentially oriented training for mental health practitioners. *Journal of Contemporary Psychotherapy, 8*, 57–68.

Goldberg, C. (1980). *In defense of narcissism*. New York: Gardner.

Goldberg, C. (1990a). The role of existential shame in the healing endeavor. *Psychotherapy, 27*, 591–599.

Goldberg, C. (1990b). *On being a psychotherapist*. Northvale, NJ: Jason Aronson.

Goldberg, C. (1990c). Typical mistakes of the seasoned practitioner. In E. Margenau (ed.) (pp. 785–798), *The encyclopedic handbook of private practice*. New York: Gardner.

Goldberg, C. (1991). *Understanding shame*. Northvale, NJ: Jason Aronson.

Gould, R. (1978). *Transformations*. New York: Simon and Schuster.

Greben, S. (1975). Some difficulties and satisfactions inherent in the practice of psychoanalysis. *International Journal of Psychoanalysis, 56*, 427–434.

Greben, S. (1984). *Love's labor: My twenty-five years in psychotherapy*. New York: Schocken.

Greenson, R. R. (1966). That "impossible" profession. *Journal of the American Psychoanalytic Association, 14*, 9–27.

Groesbeck, C. J., & Taylor, B. (1977). The psychiatrist as wounded healer. *American Journal of Psychoanalysis, 37*, 131–139.

Haigh, G. V. (1967). Psychotherapy as interpersonal encounter. In J. F. T. Bugental (ed.), *Challenges of humanistic psychology*. New York: McGraw-Hill.

Heath, D. (1991). *Fulfilling lives*. San Francisco: Jossey-Bass.

Henry, W. E., Sims, J. H., & Spray, S. L. (1971). *The fifth profession: Becoming a psychotherapist*. San Francisco: Jossey-Bass.

Henry, W. E., Sims, J. H., & Spray, S. L. (1973). *Public and private lives of psychotherapists*. San Francisco: Jossey-Bass.

Hilton, J. (1960). *Lost horizon*. New York: Pocket Books.

Jacoby, R. (1983). *The repression of psychoanalysis*. Chicago: University of Chicago Press.

Jacques, E. (1965). Death and the mid-life crisis. *International Journal of Psychoanalysis, 46*, 502–514.

Jaspers, K. (1957). *Socrates, Buddha, Confucius, Jesus*. New York: Harcourt, Brace and World.

Jones, E. (1961). *The life and work of Sigmund Freud*. Vol. III. New York: Basic Books.

Jung, C. (1956). *Symbols of transformation*. New York: Pantheon Press.

Jung, C. (1989). *Memories, dreams and reflections* (A. Jaffe, ed.). New York: Random House.

Kelly, E. L., Goldberg, L. R., Fiske, D. W., & Kilowski, J. (1978). Twenty-five years later. *American Psychologist, 33*, 746–755.

Kelly, G. (1963). *A theory of personality*. New York: Norton.

Levinson, D. J., et al. (1978). *The seasons of a man's life*. New York: Ballantine.

Lifton, R. J. (1986). *The nazi doctors*. New York: Basic Books.

Lindner, R. (1954). *The fifty minute hour*. New York: Bantam Books.

Maeder, T. (1989, Jan.). Wounded healers. *Atlantic Monthly*, 37–47.

Marmor, J. (1953). The feeling of superiority: An occupational hazard in the practice of psychotherapy. *American Journal of Psychiatry, 110*, 370–376.

Marmor, J. (1968). The crisis of middle age. *Psychiatric Forum, 29*, 17–21.

May, R. (1977, April). Freedom, determinism and the future. *Psychology*, 6–9.

Mccarley, T. (1975). The psychotherapist's search for self-renewal. *American Journal of Psychiatry, 132*, 221–224.

Neugarten, B. L. (1965). Developmental view of adult personality. In J. Birren (ed.), *Relations of development and aging*. Springfield, IL: Thomas.

Nietzsche, F. (1887). *On the genealogy of morals*. New York: Vintage. 1967.

Oberndorf, C. P. (1953). *History of psychoanalysis in America*. New York: Grune and Stratton.

Reik, T. (1964). *Listening with the third ear*. New York: Farrar, Straus and Giroux.

Rogers, C. (1975). In retrospect: Forty-six years. In R. Evans, *Carl Rogers: The man and his ideas*. New York: Dutton.

Sekaran, U., & Hall, D. T. (1989). Asynchronism in dual-career and family linkages. In M. B. Arthur, D. T. Hall, & B. S. Lawrence (eds.), *Handbook of career theory*. New York: Cambridge University Press.

Sexton, A. (1977). In L. G. Sexton & L. Amel (eds.), *Self-portrait in letters*. Boston: Houghton Mifflin.

Solomon, R. C. (1977). *The passions*. New York: Anchor Books.

Sonnenberg, S. (1991). The analyst's self-analysis and its impact on clinical work. *Journal of the American Psychoanalytic Association, 39*, 687–704.

Sontag, S. (1964). *Against interpretation*. New York: Delta Books.

Spuviell, V. (1984). The analyst at work. *International Journal of Psychoanalysis, 65*, 13–30.

Storr, A. (1983). An unlikely analyst: Marie Bonaparte. *New York Times Book Review*, Feb. 6, 1983.

Thomas, H. F. (1967). An existential attitude in working with individuals and groups. In J. F. T. Bugental (ed.), *Challenges of humanistic psychology*. New York: McGraw-Hill.

Tolstoy, L. (1960). *The death of Ivan Illyich and other stories*. New York: Signet Classics.

Valliant, G. E. (1977). *Adaptation to life*. Boston: Little, Brown.

Warkentin, J., Johnson, N. L., & Whitaker, C. (1951). A comparison of individual and multiple psychotherapy. *Psychiatry, 14*, 415–418.

Warkentin, J., & Valerius, E. (1975). Why therapy for the mature therapist. *Voices, 11*, 50–51.

Weiner, M. (1990). Older psychiatrists and their psychotherapeutic practice. *American Journal of Psychotherapy, 44*, 44–49.

Welt, S. R., & Herron, W. G. (1990). *Narcissism and the psychotherapist*. New York: Guilford.

Wheelis, A. (1956). The vocational hazards of psychoanalysis. *International Journal of Psychoanalysis, 37*, 171–184.

Wheelis, A. (1960). *The seeker*. New York: New American Library.

Wheelis, A. (1987). *The doctor of desire*. New York: Norton.

Whitehorn, J. C. (1960). Studies of the doctor as a crucial factor for the prognosis of schizophrenic patients. *International Journal of Social Psychiatry, 6*, 1960.

Winnicott, D. W. (1960). Counter-transference. *British Journal of Medical Psychology, 33*, 17–21.

Wolfenstein, M. (1966). Goya's dining room. *Psychoanalytic Quarterly, 35*, 47–83.

Yeats, W. B. (1957). "A choice." In P. Allt & R. Alspach (eds.), *The variorum edition of the poems of W. B. Yeats*. New York: Macmillian.

INDEX

NAME INDEX

SUBJECT INDEX